COGNITIVE NEUROPSYCHOLOGY
AND CONVERSATION ANALYSIS IN APHASIA
AN INTRODUCTORY CASEBOOK

COGNITIVE NEUROPSYCHOLOGY AND CONVERSATION ANALYSIS IN APHASIA

AN INTRODUCTORY CASEBOOK

Ruth Lesser and Lisa Perkins
Department of Speech,
University of Newcastle upon Tyne

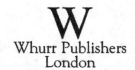

Whurr Publishers
London

© 1999 Whurr Publishers Ltd
First published 1999
by Whurr Publishers Ltd
19b Compton Terrace
London N1 2UN
England

Reprinted 2001, 2003 and 2004

British Library Cataloguing in Publication Data
A catalogue record for this book is available from the British Library.

ISBN 1 86156 068 0

Contents

Acknowledgements

We should like to express our gratitude to the people with aphasia who allowed themselves to become our 'cases', and to their families. Our thanks go also to Susan Clark, who gave us data on one of her patients and commented on our interpretations, and David Howard, for his advice on statistics and supplying the Table in Appendix A. One of us (LP) was supported by ESRC Grant number 000236456.

Introduction

Something of a sea change has taken place in aphasia therapy over the last decade. Therapists aiming to help those who have suffered brain damage, from stroke or other cause, which has resulted in impaired language, now have two new paradigms on which to draw as bases for their therapy. The first is psycholinguistic modelling as used by the recently developed discipline of cognitive neuropsychology (CN). The second is the adoption of the ethnomethodological principles of conversation analysis (CA). Psycholinguistics and CN are disciplines in their own rights, the first relating to the psychology of language in (essentially) normal users of language, and the second to the effects of brain damage on various aspects of cognitive processing. The subsection of CN which relates to aphasia, however, has adopted psycholinguistics as one of its analytic procedures. For convenience, therefore, in this workbook we use the terms 'psycholinguistic' and 'cognitive neuropsychological' interchangeably.

The aim of this workbook is to demystify these developments in aphasia therapy. We hope to show, through a series of case presentations, how they can be applied productively by speech and language therapists who work with people with aphasia, as well as by student therapists. We hope that the book will also provide some illumination for other professionals, such as clinical linguists, clinical psychologists, neurologists, neuropsychologists and therapists allied to medicine who are involved with brain-damaged patients.

The cases described are actual cases, seen by the authors or their colleagues, sometimes with students working under their supervision. They are, therefore, offered as learning exercises rather than ideal models. In putting them together we have realised how we might have improved our practice, but we describe them as they happened, to provide a learning model for other therapists struggling in similar circumstances, who we hope will be as much encouraged by discovering our faults as the merits of the system we are trying to advocate.

We have taken a very limited perspective on the cognitive neuropsychological (psycholinguistic) approach. We have restricted the analysis entirely to the processing of single words. Within this model we have also looked primarily at the processing of nouns. We have put most emphasis on auditory comprehension and speech. These are the most relevant aspects for conversational interaction, although we have used reading comprehension and writing in some cases to test for the supramodal nature of the hypothesised disorder. The psycholinguistic model we have employed is, therefore, of the simplest kind. Despite their relevance to conversation, in the interests of simplicity, we have not included sentences and narrative discourse. Fortunately, for those clinicians who wish to consider analysis of what may underlie disorders of sentence comprehension and production, a very readable handbook for therapists has recently been published (Marshall, Black and Byng, 1999), which describes a number of assessments relevant to sentence-processing. It also describes the therapy that was undertaken with three cases based on analyses of the results of such assessments.

The single-word model is used in the present workbook primarily as an introduction to the method used in the CN approach, and only secondarily as an end in itself. It is also, however, the one which may be most relevant to the ubiquitous disorder in most aphasias of naming difficulties (although we acknowledge the influence of sentence structure on word-retrieval in connected speech, see in particular Whitworth, 1995). The model has consequently been associated with a number of studies of therapy, to which we refer in so far as they could provide guidelines for considering intervention in the cases we describe. To balance the limitations of the context-free CN approach, we then discuss CA, thus making a large leap to connected speech in a social context.

We should also like to emphasise that in this workbook most of the time is spent on assessments, with their associated implications for intervention, rather than on the therapy that was actually undertaken. This is because we wish to avoid implying that CN or CA assessment dictates the use of a specific therapy. The decisions regarding the form that intervention took with an individual were influenced by a large number of factors in addition to the findings from the assessments presented here. These included the individual's level of motivation, his or her own priorities for therapy, the support available for home practice, and the length and intensity of intervention that the therapist was able to offer. In addition, several of the cases also had impairments in sentence-processing, reading and writing, which we have not explored here, but which influenced the therapy undertaken. We have therefore confined the sections on therapy to suggestions that illustrate how the assessment results presented, and the inferences drawn from them, can be used to develop targeted therapy.

We must also stress that this is intended to be a *work*book. It requires the active involvement of the reader in working through exercises. For each of the cases a number of questions are posed, with a space for the readers to suggest their own answers, before we give our own suggestions. This format is based on a number of workshops we have given, as we shall describe shortly. For the workshops, therapists and students met in small groups or pairs, and you may wish to follow this practice as an alternative to working on your own. For this reason we have included at the end of the book extra worksheets that can be photocopied. Group work can be particularly stimulating when it comes to discussing implications for therapy.

Background

First there are some issues we must address before we can claim to be moving towards a new era of 'CN–CA'-based aphasia therapy.

Both of these two paradigms are essentially new methods of assessing and understanding the person's communication disorder (both as an impairment of the patient's language system and as a functional disability in using language in everyday life). They complement each other in that the cognitive neuropsychological approach concerns itself with language-processing within the individual as a mental construct, while the conversation analytic approach concerns itself with the interactional use of communication. The first, therefore, aligns itself with understanding the impairment, the second with examining the disability. CN is experimentally driven, in that the models on which it is based were originally derived from laboratory work on normal subjects; it therefore has a strong theoretical base. Its application produces quantifiable results, which can be measured for the extent to which they confirm the theoretical postulates or not. In contrast, CA is essentially data-driven, qualitative and descriptive rather than theoretical. It is also at a much younger stage in its application to aphasia. In Part One we expand on selected aspects of CN, and in Part Two on selected aspects of CA, as they seem relevant so far to assessment and intervention in aphasia.

In respect of both these approaches we need also to ask whether there is any direct link between their use as part of an assessment and any recommendations as to what aphasia therapists can actually do to help their patients. A number of people have claimed that what therapists do still rests on their intuitions and common sense, even though they may have undertaken these elaborate assessments (e.g. Caramazza, 1989; Hillis, 1992). We have tried to address this issue through a number of arguments (Lesser and Milroy, 1993; see also Ellis, Franklin and Crerar, 1994; Mitchum and Berndt, 1995). The aim of this workbook is to demonstrate that a link can exist, by showing it through a number of examples.

We believe that both these paradigms are highly informative for the therapist in helping decisions as to if and what remediation should be attempted. We stress, however, that the link is an indirect one, and that the therapist's understanding of the whole situation remains supreme in the decision as to what resources should be drawn on. This approach to intervention is, therefore, very far from 'cookbook'-style. The approach used in aphasia therapy is one in which assessment and intervention are continuing processes. There is no one-to-one link between diagnosis and treatment. This does not mean that treatment is based on guesswork or simple common-sense, as it may appear to the untutored eye from the simplicity of the tasks through which it is executed (such as sorting pictures or engaging in conversation). Nevertheless, it is exploratory rather than prescriptive, and we have to acknowledge freely that we still have much to learn about how aphasia therapy might work (Byng, 1995).

Much of this workbook is devoted to assessment of individual cases, particularly using the psycholinguistic methodology. This is not only because this is at present the main aspect with which therapists need to be familiar when addressing the patient's impairments. It is also because assessment is a continuous facet of the clinician's interaction with people with aphasia. This is based on forming hypotheses about the underlying disorder, through both observation and response to therapy, and revising or confirming these hypotheses as all participants' (including the family's) understanding of the disorder grows. Why is this necessary? The answer lies in the complexity of the brain, mind, language and social interactions. All of these are involved in human communication, and, although much more is now known of these through research and the development of technologies (from audiorecording to brain-imaging), our understanding of them is still fragile as an underpinning to grasping what happens when they break down following damage. We are far from knowing why it should be that some people with acquired language disorders can be shown to benefit from therapy and some apparently do not. What CN has provided is a provisional framework for examining this tricky question, and for feeding back into theory evidence about the nature of those who have responded to specific therapies and those who have not. In some cases the results have been enigmatic, with individuals of similar psycholinguistic profiles responding differently to the same type of therapy (Byng, Nickels and Black, 1994). This underlines that there are many aspects of language behaviour that defy simplicity. In acknowledgement of our ignorance, assessment and intervention must therefore be intimately cyclical rather than separated stages.

Evaluation

This leads to another question. How can we be reasonably sure that it is what we have done as therapists that has effected a change in the individuals' and/or their families' communicative behaviour? For a therapeutic service to justify itself as offering more than the sympathy and listening ear that untrained volunteers could supply, we need to demonstrate that intervention is not due to recovery which would have occurred spontaneously or the placebo effect of receiving interest from someone with the label of 'expert' (Howard and Hatfield, 1987). Here again CN can help us. If people with aphasia improve significantly and specifically on what the therapist has targeted in therapy, but not on what has not been targeted (until this in turn is tackled), we have some evidence that it is statistically probable that it is the therapy which has effected the change, provided that the untreated task was of similar difficulty to the targeted task. This is easier to demonstrate if the person is several months post-onset of the aphasia. Giving therapy during the period of substantial spontaneous recovery weakens the conclusions that can be drawn as statistically significant, since many aspects of the individual's behaviour may be changing. Nevertheless, testing whether therapy has accelerated progress in the targeted behaviour is clinically informative as to whether the therapist's hypotheses about the dysfunction were sound. How the improvement was achieved can be (and should be) considered in detail, but it still leaves us with unanswered questions as to the underlying processes in the mind and brain of the language-disordered person, and in the interactions which have achieved the change.

A psycholinguistic model, as used in CN, provides us at least with a starting point for speculating as to what processes changed in the language system of the person with aphasia, and for exploring in what processes recovery might be expected to generalise to other aspects and what might not. CA similarly provides us with a framework through which to examine the impact of the linguistic deficits of the person with aphasia on interaction and the strategies used by the interlocutors to deal with these. It is important, therefore, to use, wherever possible, a therapeutic design that will help the therapist to decide whether it is indeed the intervention that has effected the change.

There are several reviews in the literature of how this can be done, most of them using the single-case methodology which is particularly pertinent to the practising clinician (Coltheart, 1989; Willmes, 1995; Franklin, 1997) Aware of the pressures on most aphasia therapists in clinical service, we have provided, in Appendix A, a brief plan as to how evaluation of the effectiveness of a specific intervention could be integrated into clinical practice as a working system for therapists applying cognitive neuropsychological principles. It applies a simple statistical test, which can be performed without the use of a calculator, as a guideline for the therapist as to whether the planned procedure has indeed achieved its aims. Appendix A also includes a short worked example. Such designs lend themselves most easily to direct therapy for the impairment applying cognitive neuropsychological principles. To date there has been very little research investigating the use of CA in the evaluation of intervention. This may be because of inherent difficulties in quantifying the results of an analysis that is dependent on local sequential context, as we discuss in Part Two; such quantification is possible but must be used with care. Structured designs have the potential to identify the effects of intervention, whether this is directed at remediating the impairment or at developing the communicative strategies of either people with aphasia or their conversational partners.

Workshops on cognitive neuropsychological models

The basis of this book is several workshops conducted by one or both of the authors, each workshop with groups of up to 30 aphasia therapists, in the UK, Australia and Canada. These followed requests to explain and practise a compilation for assessing aphasic patients of which one of the authors was an originator, Psycholinguistic Assessments of Language Processing in Aphasia (PALPA) (Kay, Lesser and Coltheart, 1992). This was one of the first attempts to make accessible to practising therapists a comprehensive system for applying cognitive neuropsychological principles in the interpretation of individual patients' disorders (Lesser, 1995). Others referred to in the literature include the Miceli, Laudanna and Caramazza (1991) battery, cited in Miceli, Capasso and Caramazza (1994), and the psycholinguistic procedure, LeMo, with several thousand single-word items, the computerised analysis of which is described by De Bleser et al. (1997). Some other psycholinguistically based assessments have focused on one modality, such as the Johns Hopkins University Dysgraphia Battery (Goodman and Caramazza, 1985), the French Canadian Protocol for the Evaluation of Lexical Semantic Disorders (Le Dorze, 1990) and the Action for Dysphasic Adults (ADA) Comprehension Battery (ADACB) (Franklin, Turner and Ellis, 1992).

We are much indebted to the participants in the PALPA workshops for the insights they gave us into how the results of psycholinguistic analyses could be applied in therapy, and have drawn greatly on the discussions on therapy that formed the final parts of these workshops. For this reason we have referred frequently in the workbook to the PALPA system, although there are now many other procedures reported in the literature that apply similar principles. Time has also exposed the many gaps in PALPA, which therapists who have the time may wish to remedy by devising their own materials. (Examples of such gaps relevant to single-word processing are the examination of specific semantic categories, connotative meaning, picture/object perception and the effect of the age of acquisition of words; see also Kay, Lesser and Coltheart, 1996.) It is therefore the basic principles of this approach that the present workbook hopes to get across to readers, rather than the implication that the specific methods illustrated here are the only, or the complete, way to achieve the same ends. In conformity with much clinical practice we have also used for most of the cases described other types of assessments, including parts of standard clinical batteries. For the sake of completeness and ease of reference while working through the cases, all the aphasia assessments referred to are listed and described in Appendix B.

Design of the workbook

As befits its title, this is a text in which we ask the reader to participate actively. It takes the form of the description of six men and women who have had strokes and become aphasic. These are real cases with whom the authors and a close colleague have worked (initials have been changed to preserve confidentiality). Each case has been chosen for its ability to help the reader understand a distinct type of processing disorder affecting single words, although this is by no means a complete account of their psycholinguistic deficits and assets.

Each case begins with a short page of general information, such as might be obtained on first referral followed by a clinical interview or case history-taking, complemented by the therapist's own observation during this interview. Sometimes this initial procedure may have included a formal aphasia test, sometimes not. As is at present common in many UK clinics for speech and language therapy, little information on the results of brain-imaging was available; but we have included it in those few cases where it was provided. The non-systematic nature of the information given in this introductory page reflects the heterogeneity of referrals in non-specialist general hospitals and community services.

From this information we ask you, the workbook reader (as we did our workshop participants), to formulate initial hypotheses as to the nature of the person's aphasia – in practice where the nub of the main stumbling block/s may lie. We then ask you to decide what detailed assessments would be necessary to test these hypotheses. These should be restricted to what is practical and economical. As we have selected these people as having disorders that can be illuminated by the use of tasks employing single words, we have provided in Appendix B information on the assessments we actually used, although there are many others you may wish to draw on.

When you have formulated your hypotheses and selected your tasks, turn to the next page. This shows you what we selected, followed, on the next page, by the results of the tests, both quantitative and qualitative in that they report not only on the numbers but also the types of errors made. These results should enable you to map on to the figure of the model, which we have supplied, where you feel the individual's principal and subsidiary strengths and weaknesses lie. Do this, and then turn to the next page, where our own interpretation is presented with its attempted justification. If you disagree, see if you can justify your decision. You may have noticed something we missed. As our selection was the one we undertook in practice, it was circumscribed by the clinical needs of the moment, and your choice may well be better than ours. The aim is for you to understand and apply the method, and not necessarily for you to conform to what we did.

On the assumption that our interpretation is on the right lines, we next ask you to consider what therapy could be attempted. This would be an initial plan for therapy, based only on the limited information obtained so far from the assessment results and the case description. This reflects the reality of the clinical situation, where there is generally pressure to begin therapy as soon as possible rather than prolong assessment. We also ask you to consider whether any other types of assistance should be offered, including assistance to the carers. When you turn to the next page, you will find our suggestions. We have not provided details of specific interventions, but, wherever possible, have given references to published articles where procedures which could be applied in this particular case have been described and tested. You may find that we have referred to the same articles in more than one case. We have repeated the information so as to make each case stand alone as complete, in case you choose to leave intervals between studying each case.

The next stage would be to develop the assessment on the basis of the response to therapy, both as measured formally and as observed through the therapist's interactions with the person with aphasia and sensitivity to leads in his or her behaviour. Although we cannot predict these at this stage, we ask you to consider this aspect, as well as the gaps in the initial assessments that have

Table 1: Summary of workbook sheets in Part One

---

1 The case description and observation/screening notes
2 Your hypotheses as to the main processing disorders
3 Our hypotheses
4 Your selection of assessments to test the hypotheses
5 Our selection of assessments
6 The results of the assessments
7 Your interpretation of the results in terms of a psycholinguistic model
8 Our interpretation of the results
9 Your suggestions for initial therapy
10 Our suggestions for initial therapy
11 Your suggestions for developing the hypotheses, based on the results and expected response so far
12 Our suggestions for developing the hypotheses

---

been revealed, and any follow-up assessments that the results have indicated. We have provided on the next page, for each case, some suggestions as to aspects to which the therapist might be alert and wish to consider for further investigation, if they seem relevant as his or her interaction with the aphasic person and family progresses. By doing this we hope we have drawn attention to the cyclical and interactive nature of assessment and intervention. The stages of the workbook sheets are summarised in Table 1.

By the time you have worked through the first three cases, i.e. those in Part One, you should be feeling fairly comfortable with the principles of a psycholinguistic analysis at the single-word level. For the last three cases, i.e. those in Part Two, we have added the interactional dimension of CA. The psycholinguistic procedure with which these case descriptions also begin should help you to locate the nature of the language-processing impairments, and give you some preliminary ideas as to how you might expect conversation to be affected. For these cases we therefore ask you, after the psycholinguistic results are reported, to consider what conversational data you might wish to collect and what specific aspects of the data you would wish to use in the analyses. We then give our own analyses. For each of these three cases we have used information from conversations audiorecorded between the person with aphasia and a carer, and sometimes between the aphasic person and therapist as well. The conversations between the person with aphasia and a carer were obtained in as natural circumstances as possible, i.e. at home, and in the absence of the therapist so that they were as unobtrusive as possible. We are aware that in using this method we

Table 2: Summary of additional workbook sheets (after sheet 8) in Part Two

9	Your selection of conversational data and parameters for analysis
10	Our selection of conversational data and parameters for analysis
11	The results of the conversation analysis
12	Your suggestions for initial therapy, based on the psycholinguistic interpretation and the conversation analysis
13	Our suggestions for initial therapy
14	Your suggestions for developing the hypotheses, based on the results and expected responses so far
15	Our suggestions for developing the hypotheses

lost some of the information that videotape recording would have given us, but the choice of audiotape was deliberate in being the most practical method available to most therapists. We then ask you to consider what implications for intervention can be drawn from the psycholinguistic impairments and conversational features for each case. You will then find our own commentary on them and our suggestions as to any implications for intervention. As in Part One, we have also added additional suggestions for developing, during intervention, the hypotheses about the nature of the individual's disorder. The workbook sheets that incorporate conversation analysis, and are added after sheet 8, are summarised in Table 2.

Before you start on your part of the workbook in Part One, make sure you are familiar with the section on the psycholinguistic model. In this section we have restricted ourselves to describing the model, the deficits that may arise from impairments of the modules and processes that comprise it, and the tests that might give more information about what is impaired and what is functioning well. We have not discussed the theory that lies behind it, since there are statements and fuller descriptions in a number of texts, such as Ellis and Young (1988) and Lesser and Milroy (1993). Nor have we discussed the criticisms that have been made of the model, e.g. that it minimises the interactive nature of processing and does not apply non-linear dynamics or a systems approach (see, for example, Seidenberg, 1988; Shallice, Glasspool and Houghton, 1997). It has a function as a working framework through which to examine some of the complexities of aphasia and make hypotheses that can be tested through therapy.

In Part Two we have discussed in more detail the principles and practice of some aspects of conversation analysis, since there are fewer texts available which are clinically relevant. We suggest therefore that you spend some time in familiarising yourself with the descriptions of CA which begin Part Two.

Part One: Applying cognitive neuropsychology

A psycholinguistic model of comprehending and producing words

This model rests on the assumption that there are separable modules for the mental processing of language. Some of these are illustrated in Figure 1. This assumption of modularity is receiving some support from studies of brain-imaging, which show increased brain activity in different areas according to the language tasks that (normal) subjects are asked to undertake while undergoing positron emission tomography (PET) or functional magnetic resonance imaging (fMRI) scans (e.g. Howard et al., 1992; Kent, 1998). The potential application of neuroimaging to the theory of aphasia therapy has been discussed by Carlomagno et al. (1997).

When we hear or read a word, or see an object whose name we know, there are early stages of analysis to be undertaken which are specific to each modality. In aphasia, unless it is accompanied by generalised cognitive impairment or a specific visual agnosia, the chief candidates for investigation are what we have called phonological and orthographic analyses. It is worth pausing to note, however, that there may be subtle disturbances of visual recognition in some aphasic people (as in one of the cases we shall be describing). The examination of people with visual processing deficits has received much attention; see, for example, the case study of John by Humphreys and Riddoch (1987) and of GK by Gilchrist, Humphreys and Riddoch (1996). The latter propose a model in which visual perception is achieved through a feature array, which results in structural units (sometimes called a structural description). These structural units are acted on in a mutually interactive way by the object recognition system and an attentional system. The examination of deficits in object perception or recognition, however, goes beyond the scope of this workbook, although we will refer later to the possible distinction between (visually accessed, non-verbal) object concepts and semantics as part of language.

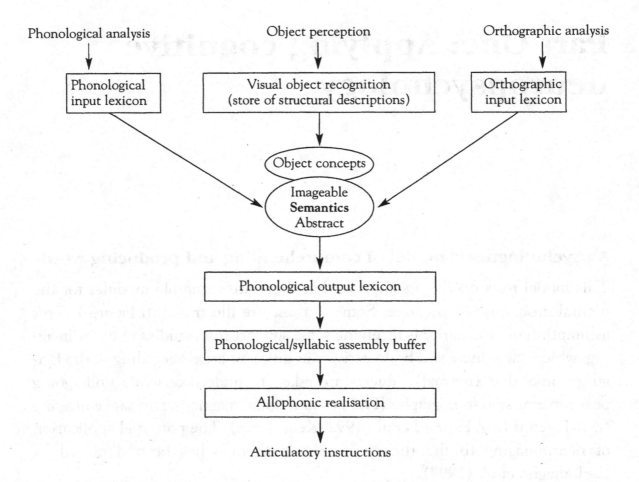

Figure 1: Listening, looking, reading and speaking for meaning

Processes in auditory comprehension

As Figure 1 shows, three stages are proposed in listening for meaning. The first is phonological analysis of the string of sounds heard. The second is recognition of the word as a familiar one that has been heard many times before and is therefore available in the 'phonological input lexicon' or store of heard words. From here, semantics has to be accessed, and the word processed for meaning.

Failure to achieve phonological analysis can result in the symptom of *word-sound deafness* (see, for example, Franklin, 1989, for a psycholinguistically based description). This will affect all later stages of auditory verbal comprehension, although not necessarily the ability to discriminate between non-verbal sounds, such as different kinds of bells. It will also mean that words cannot be echoed in repetition tasks, since a failure in this critical first stage would block access to the phonological input lexicon for repeating familiar words, either through

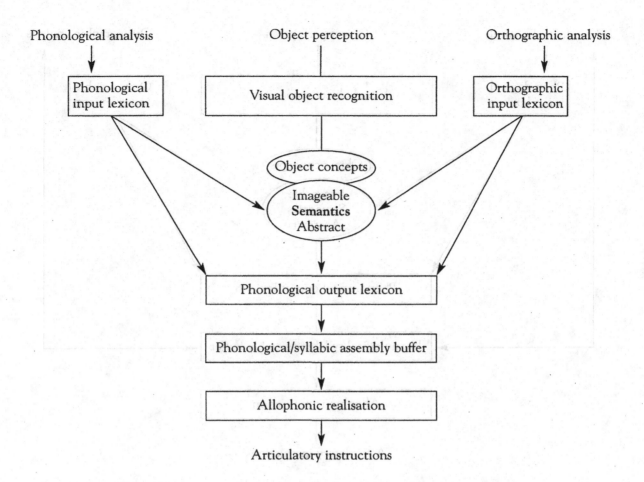

Figure 2: Repeating and reading aloud familiar words

semantics or directly through the phonological output lexicon (see Figure 2). It would also make inoperative the direct route from phonological analysis to the phonological/syllabic assembly buffer thought to be used in repeating non-words (see Figure 3). An impairment of phonological analysis will, therefore, have a profound effect on auditory comprehension, although comprehension through reading may be intact.

Impairment of the phonological input lexicon may leave the ability to repeat non-words intact through the direct route shown in Figure 3. Words will only be repeated as if they were non-words, although very familiar ones may be recognised. A damaged phonological input lexicon will also block access to meaning, resulting in *word-form deafness* (see e.g. Franklin, 1989). Even with an intact phonological input lexicon, access from it to semantics may be disturbed. This condition has been called *word-meaning deafness* (Franklin et al., 1996). People with impairments to any of these processes may still be able to access semantics from reading.

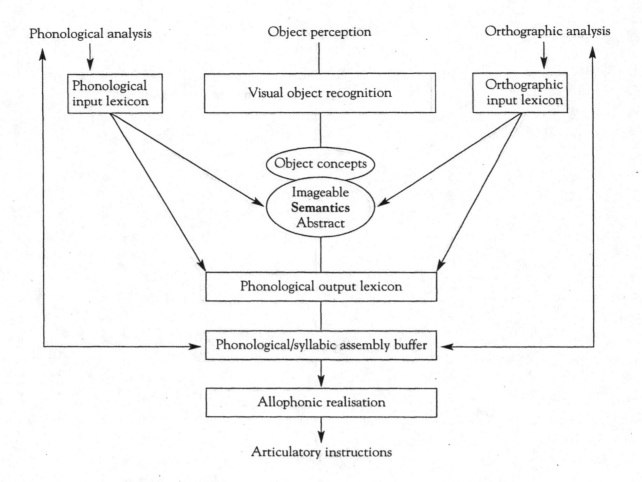

Figure 3: Repeating and reading aloud non-words

Assessing auditory comprehension

Testing any aspect of auditory verbal comprehension comes up against the possible stumbling block that the person being tested may not understand the instructions. Presenting the instructions in written form, through pictures or gesture, may help. As with other processes, auditory verbal comprehension has to be examined through a number of complementary measures, each of which may be contaminated by aspects such as short-term memory and fatigue.

PALPA 1 *Same different discrimination using non-word minimal pairs,* and ADACB P1 and P2 *Non-word minimal pairs, in different and same voices,* can be used to derive information about auditory phonological analysis. Both these assessments examine the ability to discriminate between pairs of non-words that are the same or vary by only one distinctive feature (or two in the case of ADACB), such as voicing or place of articulation. The means of testing this, however, requires the individual to keep two items in mind and make a judgement about them – two aspects that may in themselves present some difficulties for some people with aphasia. Success on the task is, therefore, more illuminating than failure; success implies that, first, the person's hearing is adequate, and second, that phonological analyses can be performed. Another way of examining auditory phonological analysis, provided that speech output processes are intact, is through repetition of non-words, as in PALPA 8 *Repetition of non-words*.

Tasks that engage the phonological lexicon by using real words include ADACB P3 *Real word minimal pairs*, PALPA 2 *Same different discrimination using word minimal pairs* and PALPA 3 *Minimal pair discrimination requiring written word selection*. The first two of these tasks are also subject to restrictions on auditory verbal memory, since two items have to be stored for comparison. PALPA 3 reduces the dependency of the response on holding two spoken items in short-term memory while making the judgement. In this task one word is spoken, and the response is to select the appropriate item from two written words. It is, however, dependent on the ability to read. All these tasks using words may be easier for people who have difficulty in dealing with non-words as such. The lexical information provided might be expected to reduce the person's reliance on phonological analysis, since it provides a context for the sounds. PALPA 4 *Minimal pair discrimination requiring picture selection*, should prove the easiest of these discrimination tasks for most people, since a semantic context is provided through the meaning of the pictures as well as a lexical one through the sound of the word. In addition, only one word has to be remembered at a time Although it includes several levels of processing, it may therefore be the task of first choice for severely impaired people with impaired spoken output.

We can obtain information related to the phonological input lexicon as such through asking people to decide whether a spoken item is a word or not – an auditory lexical decision task. This task can be performed without necessarily involving word meaning, the semantic system. ADACB L1 *Lexical decision test*, and PALPA 5 *Imageability and frequency auditory lexical decision*, provide such a task, with the words controlled for the frequency with which they occur in the language and imageability, i.e. the extent to which their referents can be visualised. (There are normative data for both word frequency and imageability, the former generally based on word counts from a large range of publications, as in, for example, Francis and Kuçera, 1982, the latter based on subjects' ratings of how easily they can visualise a picture of what the word means.) Poor performance on such tasks suggests either an impaired phonological input lexicon, or impairment of some earlier stage. More information can be gained from the type of errors that are made. An effect of frequency (i.e. low frequency words being missed more often than high frequency words) would give support to the hypothesis of impairment in the lexicon, which is assumed to be influenced by frequency. This could be tested further by other tasks that are controlled for word frequency, such as repetition in PALPA 9 *Imageability and frequency repetition*. An effect of imageability may indicate that the person is drawing on the semantic system in making the decision, and one might expect to find signs of a similarly compromised semantic system when it is examined more directly through the semantic tasks we describe shortly. As we show in Figure 2, repetition of words does not necessarily implicate semantic processing. As is indicated in the figure it is postulated that words can be repeated by a direct route from the phonological input lexicon to the phonological output lexicon, without their meaning being activated.

Semantics

Various ideas have been put forward as to the nature of the semantic system for words. Neuropsychological evidence supports a distinction between abstract and imageable items. It is common to find people with aphasia who experience more success with words of high imageability than low, possibly related to their drawing on relatively intact right hemispheres after their left hemisphere damage (Code, 1987). There is also some evidence in support of semantics being organised according to categories, which may be linked with functional use or evolutionary utility (Caramazza, 1998). As we have shown in the figures, there may also be a distinction between (visual) object concepts and language-based semantics. For a justification of this viewpoint see Davidoff and De Bleser's (1993) review of optic aphasia, which argues that visual naming of objects is possible without the use of semantics. Support for this distinction is also derived from observations of people who can perform pairing tasks that involve understanding object meaning, but who have difficulty with verbal semantic tasks.

Assessing semantics

Knowledge of object concepts can be examined through a task such as the Pyramids and Palm Trees Test (Howard and Patterson, 1992) in its picture version. Here, people are asked to select from a pair of pictures one which 'goes with' a third picture, e.g. to match a palm tree rather than a pine tree with a pyramid. It should be possible to perform this task well from knowledge of object concepts and world knowledge, without necessarily involving word semantics. (This test also has other versions, which use words or combinations of words and pictures.)

There are a number of tasks that can be used to assess word semantics. One is to present the individual with a picture, and see if a semantically related word is accepted as a correct name for it. Using this principle ADACB S2 and S2Wr *Spoken word–picture matching* and *Written word–picture matching*, are word–picture matching tests that include semantic distractors (as well as phonological). The PALPA tasks are a little different in that they include semantic, visual and semantic-visual distractors. PALPA 47 *Spoken word–picture matching*, and PALPA 48 *Written word–picture matching*, are auditory and reading versions respectively, which require the person to select a target word from five pictures; two of these are semantic distractors, close or distant, one is a visually related distractor as noted above, and one is a distractor unrelated to the target, although related to one of the other distractors so as to minimise its isolation. Half of the close semantic distractors also have visual resemblances to the target, i.e. are visual-semantic distractors, in order to test whether there is an interactive perceptual component to the semantic deficit. A central semantic impairment would be expected to show up in both the auditory and reading versions; major differences between them could indicate access problems from one modality only, such as word-meaning deafness, as described earlier.

These word–picture matching tasks necessarily use items of high imageability because pictures are involved. We have already noted that greater difficulty with words that are harder to picture mentally can be a feature of a semantic disorder, and this can be quantified through tasks that ask people to judge whether two words mean the same thing or not, using words that are controlled for imageability. In a listening version (PALPA 49 *Auditory synonym judgements*, ADACB S1 *Synonym judgements*) this requires holding two words in memory. For people with impaired auditory verbal memory, the reading version (PALPA 50 *Written synonym judgements*, ADACB S1Wr *Written synonym judgements*) may therefore prove easier. We should also be able to detect a semantic impairment from naming and spontaneous speech through word-finding failures, the production of frequent uncorrected semantic paraphasias (such as saying 'peach' instead of 'pear') and, more significantly, the acceptance of semantic paraphasias as being correct for target words.

Orthographic processes in reading

On the right side of Figures 1–3, orthographic analysis is thought to be a system that recognises letters as entities that are abstracted from their exact shapes. For example, it recognises the commonality between an upper case B and a lower case b. For reading non-words aloud, there is thought to be a direct route from orthographic analysis to the phonological/syllabic assembly buffer (see Figure 3). This route may also be used to read real words aloud, and seems to be used when 'regularisation' errors are made in reading aloud exceptionally spelled words, as in *surface dyslexia*. (An example of this would be reading HEAVY as /hivɪ/.) More commonly, reading words employs the orthographic input lexicon. Reading aloud does not necessarily involve meaning, and it is proposed that there is a direct route from the orthographic input lexicon to the phonological output lexicon which bypasses semantics. Reading for meaning necessarily involves the route through semantics. As with word-meaning deafness, a syndrome of *word-meaning blindness* has been proposed, in which access to semantics from an intact orthographic input lexicon seems to be impaired (Lambon Ralph, Sage and Ellis, 1996).

Assessing orthographic processes

One way to test whether the ability to undertake orthographic analysis is retained in people with a reading disorder is to ask them to match upper and lower case letters, as in PALPA 19 *Letter discrimination, upper to lower case matching* or PALPA 20 *Letter discrimination, lower to upper case matching*. People who have another kind of difficulty in orthographic analysis, which does not allow them to move rapidly to the orthographic input lexicon, and are described as 'letter-by-letter' readers, can be identified by use of a task such as PALPA 29 *Oral reading, letter length*, which increases the number of letters to be read in monosyllabic words from three to six. Reading will deteriorate as word length increases.

As with the phonological input lexicon, the integrity of the orthographic input lexicon can be tested through a lexical decision task, a task which does not necessarily involve semantics. PALPA provides a range of these. PALPA 24 *Visual lexical decision, legality* is an easy version where the non-words are ones that use combinations of letters which do not occur in English, like RSDO, and which are difficult to pronounce. The real words used here are also controlled for regularity of pronunciation, e.g. irregular ones like WAND, which could be pronounced /wand/ by someone unfamiliar with English, compared with MIST, which only has one possible pronunciation. Although this task does not require people to read aloud, an effect of regularity on this task would indicate that the orthographic input lexicon may be damaged, and that lexical decisions have been based on a route direct from orthographic analysis to the phonological/syllabic assembly buffer for subvocal rehearsal (see Figure 3). Corroboration of this could be found through use of PALPA 27 *Visual lexical decision, regularity*, which compares pronounceable non-words with words controlled for regularity. Further information as to the status of the orthographic input lexicon may be obtained through a test of visual lexical decision, which, like the auditory lexical decision task described above, is controlled for frequency and imageability (PALPA 25 *Visual lexical decision, imageability and frequency*). If an effect of imageability is found in this reading task, as well as in the auditory task, it is some confirmation of an involvement of the supramodal semantic system.

The link between the orthographic input lexicon and semantics can be examined without requiring a spoken response, through matching a heard word with a written one, as in PALPA 52 *Spoken word–written word matching*. The distractors here are either ones which are visually related to the target (e.g. PASTURE and PASTIME) or semantically related (e.g. HUT and SHED). Definition of homophones is another means of testing whether meaning is being accessed from the orthographic input lexicon. PALPA 38 *Homophone definition × regularity* uses words like STEEL and SCENE, which sound like STEAL and SEEN, and therefore cannot be differentiated from their pair by relying on sound (i.e. by accessing the items directly in the phonological output lexicon) rather than by linking their spelling with meaning through the orthographic input lexicon.

Processes in spoken production

Reading aloud, of course, uses other processes than those required simply for reading for making judgements such as lexical decision. This brings us to the lower parts of Figures 1–3. Output from semantics reaches the phonological output lexicon and the phonological/syllabic assembly buffer in which the putative phonemes and syllables are selected and ordered. The assembly buffer receives inputs from both the phonological output lexicon and the non-word routes used in repeating and reading, and allows some time for the preparation and ordering of the sequence of phonemes and syllables that the word or non-word requires. The final output of instructions to the articulators is preceded by preparations in which the putative phonemes and syllables assembled in the buffer are given their allophonic form, e.g. as a 'dark' or 'light' /l/.

Assessing spoken production

The principal means of examining spoken production for single words is through naming, either to definition or picture naming. Semantics, the phono-

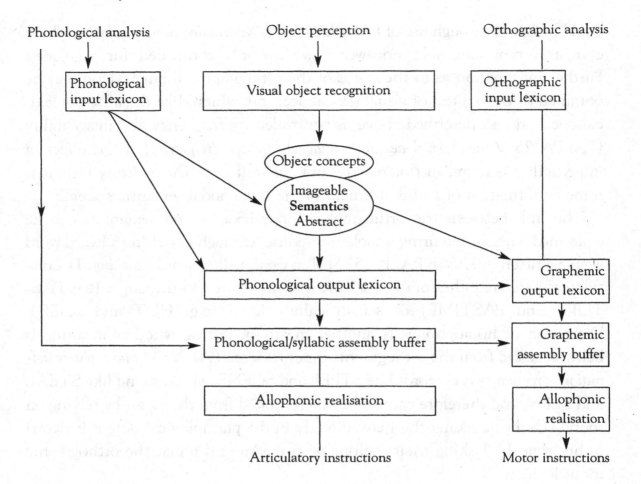

Figure 4: Naming through writing, and writing words to dictation

logical output lexicon, the assembly buffer and allophonic realisation can all be involved in the production of words spontaneously, and in naming to definition, picture naming, reading aloud and repetition. Analysis of the level of the production disorder is supported by observations of the types of behaviours and errors involved. There may be difficulty in accessing the correct item in the phonological output lexicon from semantics; people with this kind of difficulty may be helped by phonemic cueing, and should be able to repeat the word they are seeking if they hear it (the complete cue). A disorder that primarily affects the phonological output lexicon may result in the retrieval of word fragments and circumlocutions that show that the person knows what he or she wants to say. Word frequency may be particularly critical for the phonological output lexicon. A picture-naming test such as PALPA 54 *Picture naming × frequency*, which is controlled for frequency, may help to quantify this. A disorder which involves phonological/syllabic assembly would not be expected to show the influence of word frequency, although it would of length. We would expect people with this difficulty to produce a number of phonemic paraphasias whatever word production task they were asked to perform, including repetition.

As the phonological/syllabic assembly buffer is necessarily affected by length, one way of testing the influence of this would be to use PALPA 30 *Oral reading, syllable length*, a test of reading aloud which uses five-letter words that increase in number of syllables from one to three. Homophone decision, as in PALPA 28 *Homophone decision*, where people are asked to judge whether exceptionally spelled words like QUAY and KEY sound the same, provides a means of testing whether the phonological output lexicon is accessed from the orthographic input lexicon in reading aloud. The regular words in this task, e.g. PRAY and PREY, could of course be assembled for pronunciation through the route used for non-words, and an effect of word regularity would indicate a possible impairment of the orthographic input lexicon, or later stages in the lexical route. Decision tasks like these again require two words to be held in the buffer for long enough for a judgement to be made. This may present some difficulties for people with limited processing abilities.

Processes in written production

So far we have considered only spoken production of words. The model also includes the production of words through writing (see Figure 4).

Here we have a graphemic output lexicon, which comprises abstract representations of written word forms. It is closely linked with the orthographic input lexicon, and receives inputs from semantics and the phonological output lexicon – the latter may account for the uncertainties we may have in writing homophones like 'their' and 'there'. According to the model, the graphemic output lexicon feeds down to the graphemic assembly buffer, which is also thought to receive inputs from the phonological/syllabic assembly buffer. Allographic realisation includes the resolution of whether capital or lower case letters are to be used, what form of script etc.

Written naming of pictures necessarily uses a route through semantics. Writing words to dictation would normally be expected to be achieved through mediation by semantics, but the existence of patients who can spell irregular words without understanding their meaning suggests that there is a direct route which bypasses semantics, and goes from the phonological input lexicon to the graphemic output lexicon. If people consistently misspell exceptionally spelled words in dictation as if they were regular, as in surface dysgraphia, they are presumed to be using a route which takes them direct from phonological analysis to the graphemic assembly buffer, with the implication that the graphemic output lexicon cannot be reliably used.

Assessing written production

The two main means of assessing written output are through dictation and naming by writing. An effect of word frequency in spelling to dictation implicates one or other of the lexicons, the phonological input, the phonological output or the graphemic output lexicons. We might wish to quantify this through use of a test such as PALPA 40 *Spelling to dictation, imageability × frequency*. Because this task is controlled for imageability, it may give additional information as to the involvement of the semantic system. Impaired graphemic assembly may result in longer words having more errors per number of letters than shorter words, and this could be investigated through PALPA 39 *Spelling to dictation, letter length*. Provided that the person can repeat non-words well, to explore graphemic assembly we could also use PALPA 45 *Spelling to dictation, non-words*, in which non-words of three to six letters in length are given through dictation. It is useful to remember to test spelling through asking the person to spell aloud as well as in writing, since these two abilities can be dissociated (Lesser, 1990).

Practice in applying the model

When all appropriate investigations have been undertaken, it should be possible to map out on a diagram of the model which processes seem to be usable and which are impaired for an individual. This is what we shall be asking you to do in this workbook. If you would like some practice first, you might like to look at a paper by Barry (1996). This presents a fictional patient with word-finding difficulties who can repeat words but not non-words, and who produces regularisations when reading irregular words aloud, etc. The reader is supplied with the model, and asked to identify which processes are 'abolished, partially impaired or preserved'; Barry then supplies the answers.

Implications of cognitive neuropsychology for therapy for the impairment

Assessing the abilities and impairments of a person with aphasia using the single-word processing model described above gives us a very limited picture of the person's disorder. Nevertheless, the ability to use words is a key component in communication, and directly addressing a difficulty with words may be an appropriate starting point for therapy. Such therapy is sometimes described as deficit-focused. In the sense that therapy may be aimed at strengthening a weakened skill, either by exercises or by putatively enrolling undamaged brain tissues to perform the same processes, this description may be appropriate. Much of therapy, however, is aimed at helping the individual to achieve the same ends by using new means and strategies. It is therefore as useful to consider assets as much as deficits in devising therapy aimed at overcoming impairments.

There is a growing literature which reports on therapy based on a psycholinguistic model. This has been summarised in, for example, Lesser and Milroy (1993) and Lesser (1993), and we refer readers to these reviews rather than repeating them here. To illustrate the development of therapy from the implications of cognitive neuropsychological assessment, we will limit our comments to summaries of two recently published reports concerned with applying psycholinguistic principles in the remediation of anomia.

The first study (Greenwald et al., 1995) reports a detailed psycholinguistic analysis. It attempted to contrast different types of treatment within two cases, a man and a woman, both with multiple impairments including anomia. Both had difficulty in matching semantic associates using pictures (a visual-semantic impairment), and were also thought to have difficulty in activating lexical phonology from semantics. Greenwald and her colleagues devised a programme of therapy aimed first at treating the latter difficulty in both individuals. The intention was to train them to 'use a phonological cueing hierarchy as a compensatory strategy to aid lexical retrieval' (p. 28). This therefore claimed to be a strategy-teaching therapy, rather than one aimed at restituting a damaged function by practice. It should therefore generalise to untrained names, accessed through both pictures and reading. It consisted of asking the individuals to name to definition, and supplying them with increasing phonological cues until they repeated the whole word. Both improved significantly by the end of 20 sessions. They also seemed to be using the therapist's cueing hierarchy themselves, i.e. to have internalised the cueing strategy, showing some generalisation to untreated words. The second programme for both people addressed another difficulty they had in naming, i.e in visual-semantic processing using pictures. This used a semantic cueing hierarchy, in which category information ('it's an animal') and visual information ('it has a hump') were supplied. There was significant improvement with this method, and again some evidence that both individuals had spontaneously internalised the technique. No generalisation occurred, however, to a task of picture-matching using semantic associates which had not been the subject of training, perhaps because this required the simultaneous processing of four pictures. It is also possible that only the semantic representations of the treated items had improved, through reactivation/reteaching rather than the application of a relay strategy through self cueing.

The second study we describe also used a cueing technique, and drew on the psycholinguistic model in a more critical way, suggesting modifications to it based on the results of the study. Best and colleagues (1997) worked with a 62-year-old man, JOW, now living in residential accommodation after a stroke. His auditory phonological analysis and auditory lexicon functioned well, and he scored near ceiling on semantic tasks using pictures (PALPA 47 and 48). His naming was influenced by imageability but not by frequency, and was characterised by semantically linked perseverations and a sudden drop in performance after the first few items (a serial position effect). He benefited from initial phoneme cues and letter cues, particularly when these were provided in written form. Three lines of evidence led to the hypothesis that his breakdown was at a lexical semantic level: the influence of imageability and operativity (a measure based on how easily the item could be handled, etc.) on helping naming; his error types being predominantly of 'no response', with improved naming when semantic information was supplied; and the fact that his perseverations showed semantic relationships to the target.

The therapists undertook an exploratory pilot investigation of a range of different therapy procedures. Following this they conducted a controlled study comparing lexical and semantic therapy for him. In lexical therapy JOW was shown a picture and asked to write the name, if necessary by looking at the back of the picture where the name was written. In semantic therapy JOW was given a picture with four semantically related written names on the back, and asked to underline the correct one. Reassessment following the lexical therapy showed no benefit, but there was a significant improvement after the semantic therapy, which generalised to other items, but was lost a month later.

As JOW was responsive to phonemic cueing, a second study used a computerised cueing aid with nine letters on the keyboard keys; when a key was pressed the corresponding phoneme was heard. The pictures used had names which JOW found hard (50), easy (50), used letters not on the keys (32) or were not to be treated in the therapy programme (50). Over five hour-long sessions JOW practised with (and later without) the aid, pressing the initial letter and naming the picture from the cue, with the help of a therapist if needed. There was a dramatic improvement in the number of items named without help, which was maintained 15 months later. There was also generalisation to untreated pictures, and to pictures whose names began with letters not on the keys. The serial position effect had disappeared. Best and her colleagues concluded that the treatment had allowed JOW to use orthographic information he already had available to aid spoken word-finding; this was supported by the observation that his spoken naming had improved to the same degree as the success he had previously had in writing initial letters correctly. This therefore could be interpreted not as a reactivation therapy, but as one using a compensatory internalised relay. Samples of connected speech were also judged to have shown improvement by eight 'blind' therapists.

From their results, Best et al. confirm a distinction between conceptual semantics and lexical semantics, the latter being proposed as the location of the deficit in JOW's processing. They also make an amendment to the 'standard' model we have described, interpreting their results as showing that feedback occurs from the phonological assembly buffer back up to the phonological output lexicon, and perhaps back up to lexical semantics. In addition they point out that their results are more consistent with a 'cascade' model. In a cascade model, selection at one stage is not completed before activation passes on to the next stage (as it would be in a serial model), but a number of possibilities are concurrently activated until one reaches threshold through receiving some other additional input. This study is one example of how feedback from therapy can be used to test and develop the model, and indeed provide further hypotheses for testing. Given the limited explanations we have of any of the processes in the model, this feedback from therapy has the potential to play a major role in increasing our understanding, and indeed in rethinking the model if it does not fit. What people with aphasia actually do provides an excellent basis for testing theory.

Apart from the clinically focused studies which we have just outlined, there is another way in which mapping out disorders on a psycholinguistic model may help, and that is by clarifying the nature of the disability for the person with aphasia and his or her carers. This requires more than the standard general advice available in published leaflets, but an individually tailored report based on the individual's own results. A pioneering attempt at this is reported in Lesser and Algar (1995), in which simple diagrams were put into booklets that showed which processes were thought to be difficult for that particular individual, following analysis of the naming disorder. (Extracts from conversations between patient and carer were also included, to demonstrate how the psycholinguistic impairment impacted on communication – but more of that later.) To reduce the clinical time needed for preparing individual booklets, kits of sheets illustrating specific deficits can be obtained from Action for Dysphasic Adults (York Cognitive Neuropsychology Research Group, 1996); this allows the therapist to select the sheets which are relevant for that individual patient. A further step is now being taken in Glasgow with the preparation of computerised booklets, which should make preparation of individually relevant illustrations of processing deficits and assets even easier for the working clinician (*Personalised Advice Booklets for Aphasia* (PABA), Booth, Paterson and Wilson, 1999). All of these systems must be preceded by careful analysis through testing and observation, in order to map out the processes being used by the individual. This is what we ask you to do next, through the following three people to whom we introduce you.

Case 1
Mr AR

When you work through this case remember to read the information first and then write down your own interpretation and ideas before you turn the page to read ours.

Initial impressions

> Read through the case description and think about what the important features are that will guide your selection of assessments.

Case description

AR is a retired photographic dealer. He lives with his wife and has two grown-up children. AR and his wife are gregarious and have numerous friends and family with whom they enjoy socialising. AR has several hobbies, including golf, classical music and photography.

AR was 68 years old when he suffered a cerebrovascular accident while he was staying with friends. He was admitted to hospital with aphasia and a right-sided hemiplegia. A computerised tomography (CT) scan showed an extensive infarct in the region of the left middle cerebral artery. A week later AR had a further extension to the stroke.

Initial assessment of his speech and language demonstrated severe receptive and expressive difficulties. He did not follow commands at the single-word level, even when gestural support was provided. Speech output consisted of jargon, and there was evidence of apraxic difficulties.

Three weeks after the initial hospital admission, AR was transferred to his local hospital. At this stage there had been some improvement in mobility; he could now stand and transfer to a chair. There had been little change in the speech and language profile. He still showed no auditory comprehension of single words on formal tasks. In addition, he was not consistently able to carry out picture or real object matching tasks. AR's behaviour indicated that he was experiencing visual problems, as he frequently tried to close one eye to look at objects. His severely limited language skills, however, made further assessments of visual abilities virtually impossible. His output remained predominantly jargon, although he could occasionally read words aloud.

When AR was discharged home he was able to walk and he had regained use of his right hand. There had been little success in assessment of his visual problems because his language difficulties interfered with him being able to cooperate in assessment. His wife was bewildered by his communication difficulties. AR produced copious jargon and became frustrated and angry when his wife failed to understand what he was saying.

Your initial hypotheses

> Using the information given in the case description, consider the possible loci of impairments for AR's auditory comprehension deficit. Given the limited information that you have, you may have several tentative hypotheses (the number of spaces provided below is not intended as a guide). What is the justification for each of the hypotheses? What further information would you require to confirm or reject each of these?

If you want to keep the book unmarked, use the photocopiable sheets on pp. 232–239.

AR's difficulties compromise the

_____

Justification for this is that

_____

_____

_____

_____

_____

_____

_____

AR's difficulties compromise the

_____

Justification for this is that

_____

_____

_____

_____

_____

_____

_____

_____

_____

AR's difficulties compromise the

Justification for this is that

AR's difficulties compromise the

Justification for this is that

AR's difficulties compromise the

Justification for this is that

What other factors need to be taken into consideration in planning assessments for AR?

Our hypotheses

> When you have completed your hypotheses, compare them to our suggestions. As you can see, it is not possible to propose firm hypotheses, but tentative possibilities can guide the selection of assessments, and each assessment should contribute to the identification of the level of deficit.

AR's difficulties compromise some aspects of visual processing and this may interfere with all assessments which depend on visual input.

Justification for this is that his behaviour (with closing of one eye when being assessed) indicated difficulties in this area. In addition, he was unable to carry out matching tasks which are dependent on visual input.

AR's difficulties compromise auditory comprehension. From the information in the case description it is not possible to discern at which levels of processing this occurs. Assessment would be required which discriminated among a central semantic impairment, impaired access to the semantic system from the phonological input lexicon, an impairment of the phonological input lexicon itself or impairment in auditory phonological analysis. (You may have set these out as separate hypotheses on the preceding pages.).

Justification for this is that in formal testing he showed no auditory comprehension for the single word.

The assessments used will need to take into consideration AR's visual problems. If there has been no improvement in visual processing, the findings from assessments using pictorial input will be difficult to interpret. There is very little information provided regarding AR's reading comprehension, although he is able to read aloud some words. The effect of spoken versus written input requires investigation.

Your selection of assessments

> Now that you have some initial hypotheses about the loci of impairments, plan the types of assessment tasks that you would employ to test out your hypotheses. We have provided spaces for several assessments, but this does not mean that we expect you to use the exact number. You will find that selection of one assessment will be influenced by the potential findings of previous ones carried out.

Assessment

Justification for selection

Assessment

Justification for selection

Assessment

Justification for selection

Assessment

Justification for selection

Assessment

Justification for selection

Assessment

Justification for selection

Our selection of assessments

> Now you have selected possible assessments compare them to the suggestions that we have made. Remember that there is no single right way of assessing someone using a psycholinguistic perspective. You should, however, be able to justify the need for each of the assessments in testing out specific hypotheses regarding the locus of impairment. If you selected different assessments, look at the assessments that were selected and work out the rationale behind this choice.
>
> It is important to remember that, as discussed in Part One, psycholinguistic assessment is only one facet of the investigation. Assessment of functional ability would run in tandem with this. The information from the psycholinguistic investigation provides invaluable information for the planning of intervention focused on maximising communicative function, as it allows identification of the abilities which can be harnessed.

Assessment: Visual matching tasks (e.g. the matching subtests of the Aphasia Screening Test; Whurr, 1981).

Justification for selection: Matching tasks will allow investigation of whether there has been any resolution of AR's visual difficulties and improvement of his basic association skills. If he is able to carry out these tasks then it will be possible to continue with assessments which rely on pictorial input. If he is unable to carry out these tasks, exploration of his matching ability using touch could be investigated to check his association skills separated from visual processing difficulties.

Assessment: Single-word cross-modal tasks using both auditory and written modality will be necessary. If AR is able to carry out the visual matching task then pictures could be used. For screening, the reading and auditory comprehension subtests of the Aphasia Screening Test could be used. For more detailed investigation PALPA 47 *Spoken word–picture matching* and PALPA 48 *Written word–picture matching* could be employed. If AR is still unable to carry out matching tasks because of visual difficulties, it will be necessary to devise an assessment of single-word comprehension based on tactile input with real objects, again using both spoken and written input. Consideration of the impact of visual problems on reading will need to be considered.

Justification for selection: Comparison of AR's comprehension for auditory and written input will allow the investigation of whether his comprehension difficulty is a central semantic one, in which case he would be expected to perform equivalently in both modalities, or whether it is specific to one modality. Alternatively, he may have impairment in input processing for both spoken and written input. His pattern of errors on assessments PALPA 47 and 48 will help to narrow down the possible loci of impairment. If AR has a random error pattern on the auditory version then this will imply that the impairment could involve the phonological input lexicon or auditory phonological analysis, and further assessment of this possibility will be required. If AR has a semantic error pattern which is equivalent across both modalities, this will indicate a central semantic impairment. If he has a semantic error pattern for only one modality of input this will suggest impaired access from that modality (the phonological input lexicon or the orthographic input lexicon). His possible selection of visual distractors would point to the impact of visual difficulties.

Assessment: A lexical decision task such as PALPA 5 *Auditory lexical decision: imageability × frequency* or ADACB L1 *Lexical decision.*

Justification for selection: If AR shows a random error pattern on auditory word–picture matching, lexical decision would allow a test of the hypothesis of an impairment of the phonological input lexicon. If AR is impaired on this assessment it will also be necessary to check auditory phonological analysis.

Assessment: Auditory discrimination assessments. Possible assessments include PALPA 1 *Non-word minimal pairs,* PALPA 2 *Word minimal pairs,* ADACB P1 *Non-word minimal pairs* and ADACB P3 *Real word minimal pairs.*

Justification for selection: If AR has been shown to be impaired on lexical decision, this assessment will give some guidance as to whether this is due to an impairment to the phonological input lexicon itself or to an impairment of auditory phonological analysis.

Assessment results

> Now read through the findings of the assessments we carried out.

Aphasia Screening Test (Whurr, 1996)

Matching subtests A1 to A8: AR completed all matching tasks without error, including matching pictures to pictures, colours to colours, sentences to sentences and pictures to objects.

Reading comprehension subtests A9 to A11: AR scored 4 out of 5 on the written word–picture match. He scored 0 out of 5 on both the written sentence–picture match and the written two part commands (e.g. raise your hand). Given this performance at floor level it was not felt appropriate to test him with the longer commands of subsection A12.

Auditory comprehension subtests A13 to A17: on the selection of the following items to auditory command AR scored:

Pictures	2 out of 5	Letters	3 out of 5
Colours	4 out of 5	Written words	2 out of 5
Numbers	2 out of 5	Two part commands	0 out of 5

PALPA 47 Spoken word–picture matching

AR scored 9 out of 20 on the first half of this assessment. He made six close semantic errors, four distant semantic errors and one visual error. He was slow and reticent in carrying out the assessment, and the second half was therefore not presented.

PALPA 48 Written word–picture matching

AR scored 14 out of 20 on the first half of this assessment. He made four close semantic errors and two distant semantic errors.

PALPA 5 Auditory lexical decision: imageability × frequency

AR scored 78 out of 80 on this assessment. This is equivalent to the mean of the PALPA control subjects, so the auditory discrimination tasks were not given.

Your interpretation of the results of the assessments

> What do the assessment results mean? Map out your hypotheses as to the locus or loci of AR's comprehension deficit based on these findings, using the diagram of the model. Indicate also what processes seem to be preserved and which levels you are uncertain about from the assessment results so far. Note down the justification in support of your hypotheses.

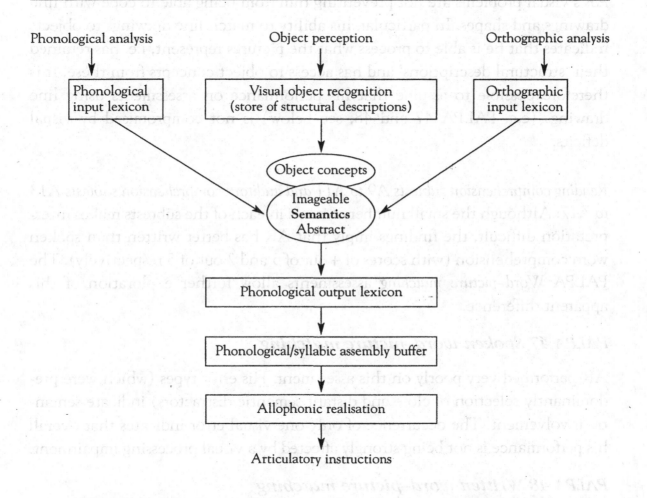

Justification for hypotheses

Our interpretation of the results of the assessments

> Now read through our interpretation of the findings.

Aphasia Screening Test

Matching subtests A1 to A8: Performance on the matching tasks indicates that AR's visual problems are not preventing him from being able to cope with line drawings and shapes. In particular, his ability to match line drawings to objects indicates that he is able to process what the pictures represent, i.e. has retained their 'structural descriptions' and has access to object concepts from these. It is therefore possible to assume that his performance on assessments using line drawings (e.g. PALPA 47 and 48, see below) is not compromised by visual deficits.

Reading comprehension subtests A9 to A11 and auditory comprehension subtests A13 to A17: Although the small number of items in each of the subtests makes interpretation difficult, the findings imply that AR has better written than spoken word comprehension (with scores of 4 out of 5 and 2 out of 5 respectively). The PALPA *Word–picture matching* assessments allow further exploration of this apparent difference.

PALPA 47 Spoken word–picture matching

AR performed very poorly on this assessment. His error types (which were predominantly selection of close and distant semantic distractors) indicate semantic involvement. The occurrence of only one visual error indicates that overall his performance is not being strongly affected by a visual processing impairment.

PALPA 48 Written word–picture matching

Performance with written input, while superior to that of spoken input (see PALPA 47), is still markedly impaired. As in the spoken version the errors were almost exclusively semantic in nature. This indicates a central semantic impairment, since errors are made for both modalities of input.

Poorer performance on the auditory version does indicate that there may be a further locus of impairment which results in a more severe deficit in the auditory modality. Possible loci include auditory phonological analysis, the phonological input lexicon or access from the phonological input lexicon to the semantic system. Is it possible to distinguish among these different loci? If the impairment involves auditory phonological analysis or the phonological input lexicon, it is not clear why these would give rise to the semantic error pattern. Problems at these levels could be expected to give a random error pattern. It has been reported in the literature, however, that impairment accessing the semantic system from an intact phonological input lexicon is influenced by semantic factors (Franklin, 1989, subject DRB).

PALPA 5 Auditory lexical decision: imageability × frequency

AR's good performance on this assessment does allow us to reject an impairment involving the phonological input lexicon. In addition, performance on this task requires preserved auditory phonological analysis. If this were impaired, one could expect errors to be made on judgements regarding the status of non-words which differ by only one phoneme from real words. The findings therefore suggest that, in addition to a central semantic impairment, AR has a further impairment in access to the semantic system from an intact phonological input lexicon.

Planning intervention

> On the basis of the interpretation of the assessment results, it has been hypothesised that AR's comprehension deficit involves a central semantic impairment compounded by impaired access from the phonological input lexicon to the semantic system. What initial approach to therapy would you derive from this?

Our suggestions for initial intervention

> Now that you have thought about some possible interventions, compare them with our suggestions. Remember that these are only tentative ideas and may very well differ from yours. Both your and our ideas may be appropriate. The important issue is that intervention should be motivated by theoretical principles.

Considering, first, impairment-focused therapy, there are numerous approaches commonly used in clinics to treat semantic impairments. These include semantic categorisation tasks, word–picture matching with distractors of increasingly close semantic relationships and selecting items to definitions. Behrmann and Lieberthal (1989) describe a reactivation therapy programme for a client with a central semantic impairment. Therapy was directed at improving comprehension of three categories (transport, body parts and furniture), with words in each category divided into treated and untreated sets. Over a period of 6 weeks, 15 hours of therapy were directed at teaching first the general features of the category and then the specific identification of its members. The programme was backed up by home assignments. There was a significant improvement on all treated sets, with within-category generalisation for untreated words for two of the three categories. There was no generalisation to two categories which had not been treated.

A number of other therapy studies have been reported for clients with a semantic impairment which compromises naming. Nettleton and Lesser (1991) applied a semantic therapy programme (consisting of word–picture matching among semantic associates, semantic judgements and category sorting) to two subjects with a hypothesised semantic impairment and two subjects with a hypothesised impairment to the phonological output lexicon. As predicted, the subjects with an impairment to the phonological output lexicon did not improve in naming after semantic therapy. For the two subjects with a semantic impairment, one showed significantly improved naming while the other showed a qualitative improvement with fewer semantic paraphasias. Marshall et al. (1990) also describe a therapy study aimed at enhancing semantic abilities for subjects with anomia as a consequence of a central semantic impairment. The therapy consisted of matching pictures to written words which were semantically related. Improvement on treated words but not untreated words was seen in naming after from 3 to 10 hours of intervention. Other efficacy studies of semantic therapy described in the literature include those by LeDorze et al. (1994), Hillis and Caramazza (1994), Lowell, Beeson and Holland (1995) and Best, Howard, Bruce and Gatehouse (1997).

AR's further impairment in access to the semantic system from the phonological input lexicon indicates that he will be more successful on all tasks with written input. It may therefore be possible to use written input to support auditory input. After practice, this could gradually be phased out so that the task is predominantly one of auditory comprehension. The severity of impairment in single-word processing indicates that it would be necessary to work at a single-word level before work at the sentence level could be considered.

In addition to direct work on the language impairments, compensatory strategies could be introduced. AR's better reading comprehension could be harnessed. For example, a communication book with information on key subjects (e.g. names of family and friends, daily activities, food, etc.) could be developed. This could be used by his wife to support auditory comprehension. In addition, while AR's expressive deficits are not the focus of discussion here, given his jargon production, both gesture and a communication book could be used as a two-way mode of communication.

Green (1982) discusses the teaching of communicative strategies, suggesting that useful ones are taught by instruction, demonstration and rehearsal in a variety of situations. Ensuring that AR's communication partners are aware of the nature of his difficulties is important in helping them to use effective strategies to enhance his comprehension. Materials to assist in this type of approach are available in the ADA advice booklets (York Cognitive Neuropsychology Research Group, 1996) and the Glasgow computer package for the preparation of individualized booklets (Booth et al., 1999) as described in Part One.

Miller (1989) discusses approaches to facilitate partners' communicative strategies using the tactic of simulating the aphasic person's predicament by placing the partner in a foreign language situation. To simulate impaired comprehension Miller suggests the use of passages and questions in which there are some recognisable or English language cues incorporated. In tackling the task, strategies that aid comprehension such as emphasising the meaning of a key word or employing a non-verbal signal through the use of a real object, a gesture or tone of voice are gradually introduced. After completion of the task, the effectiveness of cues can be discussed with the partner as well as the significance of prior information and how meanings can be inferred.

Developing the hypotheses

> Remember that the results of assessment (and of intervention) feed back into developing the hypotheses, as the assessment of AR has already shown. There may also be gaps in your interpretation, which the results have revealed. Use this page to write down what further investigations you might wish to consider to develop your hypotheses, some of which may depend on AR's response to therapy. **Cover up the next page (which has our suggestions) until you have written yours down.**

Our suggestions for developing the hypotheses

> Now read through the suggestions that we have made and compare them with your own.

AR's comprehension of gesture could be investigated, so that, providing that this was intact, his wife could be encouraged to support his comprehension using this form of communication to supplement spoken input. An assessment to consider is the New England Pantomime Recognition Test of Duffy and Duffy (1984). It may also be useful, if AR shows response to therapy for his semantic disorder, to explore any distinction made between imageable and abstract semantics.

The assessments so far have focused on input. More information could be obtained through examining output. For example, AR's naming abilities could be investigated, to establish the nature of his 'jargon' errors, and consider at what level(s) his difficulties lie. Semantic errors may be expected, but it is also possible that there may be impairment of the phonological output lexicon, the phonological assembly buffer and allophonic realisation. The first might be influenced by word frequency, and a test controlled for frequency such as PALPA 54 *Picture naming × frequency* could be used. The second might be influenced by number of syllables, and repetition or oral reading could be attempted, as in PALPA 7 *Syllable length repetition* or PALPA 30 *Syllable length reading*. Impairment of allophonic realisation might be consistent with the report in the case description that AR has apraxia of speech. Searching behaviours and the production of non-English phonemes might reveal this, but it is generally difficult to tease out such an impairment through a naming test if it coexists with other output difficulties, as hypothesised above

Some patients with jargon aphasia are thought to have difficulties in lexical retrieval, for which they compensate by producing meaningless strings of phonemes as fillers in syntactic frames (Butterworth, 1979); analysis of AR's spontaneous speech might illuminate this, and also the degree to which morphosyntactic features are retained. If the jargon is severe, it may be necessary to elicit connected speech through description of a composite picture, so that there is the possibility of detecting some target words.

Case 2
Mr RV

When you work through this case remember to read the information first and then write down your own interpretation and ideas before you turn the page to read ours.

Initial impressions

Read through the case description and think about what the important features are that will guide your selection of assessments.

Case description

RV is a 65-year-old man who had retired from a manual job at a local factory when he was 60 because of ill health. He lives with his wife; they have six grown-up children and 11 grandchildren who live locally and whom they see frequently. He is a sociable person, who regularly attends the local Working Men's Club. He also attends a local day club with his wife.

When he was 54 he had a minor stroke, which resulted in a right hemiparesis which resolved completely. There was no report of aphasia associated with this stroke, although RV reports that he had problems with writing following this episode and had not written since this time.

At the age of 65 he was admitted to hospital with an acute inferior myocardial infarction. He made a good recovery and was discharged home. Three weeks later he suffered a left cerebrovascular infarct at home, with aphasia. The consultant reported that he was otherwise neurologically intact, and he was not admitted to hospital. Six weeks later, due to the high level of anxiety that RV and his wife were experiencing, the consultant requested a speech and language assessment.

When RV and his wife attended the speech and language therapy clinic for their first visit, both were extremely distressed about the communication problems that they had been experiencing, and much of the session was spent explaining aphasia and providing reassurance. His wife reported that RV seemed not to take in what she said to him and that he had extreme difficulty telling her anything. He was getting all the names of the family muddled up despite her attempts to correct him. In the session he exhibited severe word-finding difficulties and frequently aborted his attempts to communicate.

Part of the British Shortened Version of the Minnesota Test for the Differential Diagnosis of Aphasia was adminstered, with the following results.

1. On Section A (auditory disturbance) he scored at the 23rd percentile. He recognised 4 out of 5 common words and discriminated between paired words correctly for 3 out of 5 items. He scored 1 out of 5 on recognising letters, 0 out of 5 on identifying items named serially, 3 out of 5 on understanding sentences and 2 out of 5 on understanding paragraphs (these two latter tasks require yes/no responses).

2. His naming of pictures was severely impaired, with a 0 out of 5 score, his errors comprising two unrelated responses, two semantic paraphasias and one neologism. His ability to repeat what he heard was also impaired, resulting in scores of 2 out of 5 on monosyllables and 1 out of 5 on phrases. He refused to attempt subtests which required him to write.

In conversational speech he showed a severe word-finding difficulty with neologisms, semantic paraphasias and blocks.

Your initial hypotheses

> Using the information given in the case description, consider the possible loci of RV's impairments. Given the limited information that you have, you may have several tentative hypotheses. What is the justification for each of the hypotheses? What further information would you require to confirm or reject each of these?

If you want to keep the book unmarked, use the photocopiable sheets on pp. 232–239.

RV's difficulties compromise the _____
_____

Justification for this is that _____
_____
_____
_____
_____
_____

RV's difficulties compromise the _____
_____

Justification for this is that _____
_____
_____
_____
_____
_____
_____
_____

RV's difficulties compromise the _____

_____

Justification for this is that _____

_____

_____

_____

_____

_____

RV's difficulties compromise the _____

_____

Justification for this is that _____

_____

_____

_____

_____

What other factors need to be taken into consideration in planning assessments for RV?

_____

_____

_____

_____

_____

_____

Our hypotheses

> When you have completed your hypotheses, compare them to our suggestions. As you can see, it is not possible to propose firm hypotheses, but tentative possibilities can guide the selection of assessments, and each assessment should contribute to the identification of the level of deficit.

RV's difficulties compromise auditory phonological analysis.

Justification for this is that he scored at only the 23rd percentile on the auditory disturbance section of the Shortened MTDDA assessment and his wife reports functional comprehension difficulties. While other loci of deficit could explain impaired comprehension (see hypotheses below), two factors suggest that auditory phonological analysis could be compromised. First, he performs poorly on discrimination of pairs of words which differ by only one phoneme. Second, repetition ability is compromised.

RV's difficulties compromise the phonological input lexicon or access from it to the semantic system.

Justification for this is that, as noted above, he has impaired auditory comprehension and made an error on an easy task of recognition of common words. Further assessment is required to distinguish whether this arises as a consequence of an impairment at this level or in auditory phonological analysis.

RV's difficulties compromise the semantic system.

Justification for this is that he produced semantic paraphasias in both picture naming and spontaneous speech and exhibited severe word-finding difficulties. His impaired performance on the auditory comprehension subtests may also reflect a semantic processing impairment, although further assessment is required to investigate whether this results from impaired auditory processing as discussed above.

RV's difficulties compromise the phonological output lexicon.

Justification for this is that on observation in the clinic he demonstrated a severe word-finding difficulty with blocks and neologisms. His production of semantic errors and neologisms on naming and in spontaneous speech could also reflect impaired access to the phonological output lexicon.

RV's difficulties compromise the phonological output buffer.

Justification for this is that he has impaired repetition ability, although, as highlighted above, this could also be explained as arising from impaired auditory phonological analysis.

Other factors that need to be taken into consideration in planning assessments include RV and his wife's high level of anxiety. It will be important not to ask him to undertake too much assessment and not to concentrate only on tasks which subject him to failure.

As no assessment of RV's reading comprehension is reported in the case description, it is not possible to ascertain whether he shows a modality influence in input processing. This needs to be explored. Modality influence on output processing cannot be explored as, since his earlier stroke, RV has not written and is reluctant to make any attempt at writing.

Your selection of assessments

Now that you have some initial hypotheses about the loci of impairments, plan the types of assessment tasks that you would employ to test out your hypotheses. We have provided spaces for several assessments, but this does not mean that we expect you to use the exact number. You will find that selection of one assessment will be influenced by the potential findings of previous ones carried out.

Assessment

Justification for selection

Assessment

Justification for selection

Assessment

Justification for selection

Assessment

Justification for selection

Assessment

Justification for selection

Assessment

Justification for selection

Our selection of assessments

> Now you have selected possible assessments compare them to the suggestions that we have made. Remember that there is no single right way of assessing someone using a psycholinguistic perspective. You should, however, be able to justify the need for each of the assessments in testing out specific hypotheses regarding the locus of impairment. If you selected different assessments, look at the assessments that were selected and work out the rationale behind this choice.
>
> It is important to remember that psycholinguistic assessment is only one facet of the investigation. Assessment of functional ability would run in tandem with this. The information from the psycholinguistic investigation provides invaluable information for the planning of intervention focused on maximising communicative function, as it allows identification of the abilities which can be harnessed.

Assessment: Word–picture matching assessments in both spoken and written modality. Possible assessments that could be used are PALPA 47 *Spoken word–picture matching* and PALPA 48 *Written word–picture matching* or ADACB S2 *Auditory word–picture matching* and ADACB S2Wr *Written word–picture matching*.

Justification for selection: These assessments will allow exploration of whether the auditory comprehension impairment identified on the subtests of the Shortened MTDDA and reported by RV's wife arise as a consequence of impaired semantic processing. If this is the case, performance on both auditory and written modalities will be compromised. If performance is better on the written version, this supports the hypothesis that some aspect of auditory input processing is impaired.

Assessment: Auditory discrimination assessments. Possible assessments include

PALPA 1 *Non-word minimal pairs*, PALPA 2 *Word minimal pairs*, PALPA 4 *Word minimal pairs requiring picture selection*, ADACB P1 *Non-word minimal pairs* and ADACB P3 *Real word minimal pairs*. PALPA 3 *Word minimal pairs requiring written selection* could also be used if RV's reading ability is not impaired, information on which will be gained from presenting a written word–picture matching assessment (see above).

Justification for selection: These assessments will allow exploration of auditory phonological analysis. If RV is able to make the fine discriminations required by these assessments, it will allow us to rule out impairment in auditory phonological analysis as underlying his comprehension impairment.

Assessment: Assessment of auditory lexical decision, for example PALPA 5 *Auditory lexical decision: imageability × frequency* or ADACB L1 *Lexical decision test*.

Justification for selection: If RV's performance on auditory discrimination assessments is poor, it will not be necessary to undertake this assessment, because it can be predicted that his performance will be poor on the basis of impaired auditory phonological analysis. If he performs well on these assessments, however, investigation of lexical decision will allow us to check whether he has impairment involving the phonological input lexicon.

Assessment: Picture naming assessment. Given that RV's initial assessment suggested a severe naming deficit, use of a test with reasonably high-frequency items, such as PALPA 53 *Picture naming*, will be preferable to assessments such as the Boston Naming Test or PALPA 54 *Picture naming × frequency*, which include low-frequency targets.

Justification for selection: This assessment will allow exploration of RV's output deficit and provide data for further analysis to allow us to tease out the relative contribution of impairments to the semantic system, the phonological ouput lexicon and the phonological output buffer.

Assessment results

> Now read through the results of the assessments we carried out.

PALPA 47 Spoken word–picture matching

RV scored 23 out of 40, with 10 close semantic errors, six distant semantic errors and one visual error.

PALPA 48 Written word–picture matching

RV scored 37 out of 40 with two close and one distant semantic errors.

PALPA 2 Word minimal pairs

RV scored 39 out of 72 (54%). His level of performance was equivalent for same (19 out of 36) and different (20 out of 36) pairs. He scored 6 out of 12 on initial contrasts, 5 out of 12 on final contrasts and 8 out of 12 on metathetic contrasts. He scored 5 out of 12 on voice contrasts, 6 out of 12 on manner contrasts and 8 out of 12 on place contrasts. There was a slight effect of frequency with 9 out of 18 correct for low frequency word pairs in contrast to 12 out of 18 correct for high frequency word pairs.

PALPA 3 Word minimal pairs requiring written selection

RV scored 50 out of 72 (69%). He was more impaired on final contrasts (10 out of 24) in comparison to either initial (17 out of 24) or metathetic (19 out of 24) contrasts. Performance on contrasts of voice (12 out of 18, 68%), manner (15 out of 21, 71%) and place (23 out of 33, 70%) was equivalent. The poorer performance with low-frequency items identified in PALPA 2 was replicated in this assessment, with 22 out of 36 low-frequency items correct in comparison to 28 out of 36 high-frequency items.

PALPA 53 Picture naming

RV made only 3 correct responses out of 40. Errors included failures to produce a response, perseverations on previous responses and neologisms. He frequently produced gestures to indicate recognition of the picture. Attempts to circumlocute were abandoned as he ran into word-finding difficulties in their production. When given the picture name, he was able to correctly repeat 22 out of 25 of the items.

Your interpretation of the results of the assessments

What do the assessment results mean? Map out your hypotheses of the locus or loci of RV's comprehension deficit based on these findings, using the diagram of the model. Indicate also what processes seem to be preserved and which levels you are uncertain about from the assessment results so far. Note down the justification in support of your hypotheses.

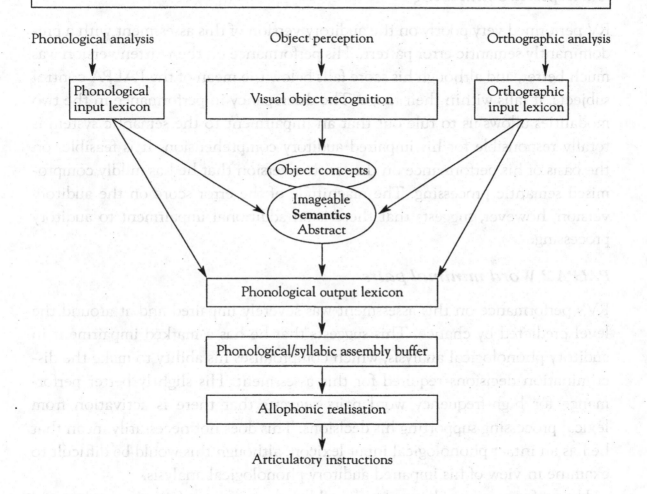

Phonological analysis   Object perception   Orthographic analysis

Phonological input lexicon   Visual object recognition   Orthographic input lexicon

Object concepts

Imageable **Semantics** Abstract

Phonological output lexicon

Phonological/syllabic assembly buffer

Allophonic realisation

Articulatory instructions

Justification for hypotheses

Our interpretation of the results of the assessments

> Now read through our interpretation of the findings.

PALPA 47 Spoken word–picture matching and PALPA 48 Written word–picture matching

RV performed very poorly on the auditory version of this assessment with a predominantly semantic error pattern. His performance on the written version was much better, and although his score falls below the mean of the PALPA control subjects, it falls within their range. The discrepancy in performance in the two modalities allows us to rule out that an impairment to the semantic system is totally responsible for his impaired auditory comprehension. It is feasible, on the basis of his performance on the written version that he has mildly compromised semantic processing. The magnitude of the error score on the auditory version, however, suggests that there is an additional impairment to auditory processing.

PALPA 2 Word minimal pairs

RV's performance on this assessment was severely impaired and at around the level predicted by chance. This suggests that he has a marked impairment in auditory phonological analysis, which compromises his ability to make the discrimination decisions required for this assessment. His slightly better performance for high-frequency word pairs suggests that there is activation from lexical processing supporting his decisions. This does not necessarily mean that he has an intact phonological input lexicon, although this would be difficult to examine in view of his impaired auditory phonological analysis.

His performance at chance level could also arise from a failure to understand the task, which is a relatively abstract one to explain to somebody with compromised comprehension. A further assessment which allows examination of auditory phonological analysis but with slightly different task demands would allow this possibility to be investigated (see below).

PALPA 3 Word minimal pairs requiring written selection

RV's performance on this assessment supports the interpretation of his performance on PALPA 2, as indicating impaired auditory phonological analysis. While his score is above that predicted by chance, he is still severely impaired on the task. His slightly better performance on this assessment in comparison to PALPA 2 may be explained by it only requiring the processing of one word in the auditory modality in comparison to two words for PALPA 2. His better performance for high-frequency words replicated the pattern observed for PALPA 2.

PALPA 53 Picture naming

RV's performance on this assessment was extremely poor. Given his relatively good performance on PALPA 48 *Written word–picture matching*, it is unlikely that an impairment to the semantic system could account for the output problems that he demonstrates. The failures to respond and the neologisms that he produced could be accounted for by impaired access to the phonological output lexicon.

His ability to repeat the majority of the words that he could not name is surprising given the indication from other assessments that auditory phonological analysis is impaired, as repetition requires this processing. In this context, however, he had the picture to provide semantic information and assist in disambiguation of the word to be repeated. In addition, he had access to lip-reading which is prevented in PALPA 2 and 3 and which is thought to help compensate for impaired auditory phonological analysis. This repetition ability indicates that processing in the phonological assembly buffer is intact enough to support repetition of the phonologically simple words of this assessment (the majority of which have one or two syllables).

Planning intervention

On the basis of the interpretation of the assessment results, it has been hypothesised that RV's comprehension deficit involves an impairment in auditory phonological analysis. The central semantic system may also be mildly impaired. In addition, spoken output is thought to be compromised by a severe impairment in access to the phonological output buffer. What initial approach to therapy would you derive from this interpretation?

Our suggestions for initial intervention

Now that you have thought about some possible interventions, compare them with our suggestions. Remember that these are only tentative ideas and may very well differ from yours. Both your and our ideas may be appropriate. The important issue is that intervention should be motivated by theoretical principles.

The cognitive neuropsychological assessment has highlighted that RV has numerous processing deficits. The high level of anxiety of both RV and his wife indicate that these deficits are having a large functional impact.

Assessment has identified that RV has impaired auditory phonological processing. This could be addressed through deficit-focused therapy aimed at reteaching/reactivating RV's ability to make phonological distinctions. The pattern of performance on PALPA 2 and 3 provides some indication of how this work could be structured. RV performed better on PALPA 3, which required processing of one word in comparison to PALPA 2, which required processing of two. Work could therefore focus on increasing RV's retention of stimuli in short-term memory. His performance was better for initial and metathetic contrasts than for final ones and better for high-frequency words. In addition, on PALPA 2 he performed better on discrimination of place contrasts. Therapy materials could be designed in a hierarchy starting from discrimination of contrasts for which he appears more reliable. Morris et al. (1996) and Morris and Franklin (1995) describe this type of therapy programme for a man with impaired auditory phonological analysis and demonstrate its effectiveness. Grayson, Franklin and Hilton (1997) describe an auditory therapy, in association with semantic and sentence therapy, in a successful evaluation study. The assessment of RV's naming ability revealed better repetition in this situation than when repetition was presented as an isolated task, and we speculated that this was because of the added input from semantics with the pictures. It could be useful to draw on this facilitation through pictures when giving phonological discrimination tasks, as does the Grayson et al. technique.

A communication-focused approach could also be taken either in conjunction with impairment-focused work or as an alternative to it.

Research has shown that lip-reading can greatly assist in auditory discriminations (Reisberg, McLean and Goldfield, 1987). The impact of lip-reading on RV's comprehension could be explored, and RV and his wife encouraged to maximise its use through ensuring eye contact and good lighting conditions when talking to each other. If impairment-focused work was also being undertaken, it would be useful to encourage RV to use visual cues to assist in discrimination to support auditory discrimination.

The discrepancy in performance on the auditory word–picture matching task with good performance with written input suggests that this relatively intact ability could be explored. RV's wife could be encouraged to write down key words to reinforce information that is important. The development of a communication booklet with written input could also be explored so that frequently used pieces of information (such as family names, food choices, times) could be readily accessed.

In addition to processing deficits which compromise auditory comprehension, RV's output was identified as being severely compromised by impaired access to the phonological output lexicon, with the production of neologisms, semantic paraphasias and frequent abandoned attempts because of failures in retrieval. While the role of auditory phonological analysis in monitoring output is not clear from the research literature, preliminary findings from a research project in progress (Buerk, Franklin and Howard, 1997) suggest that improved output is achieved with therapy targeted at improving skills in auditory phonological analysis. It may therefore be appropriate to delay any deficit-focused work on output until work on input has been completed.

Communication-focused work could, however, be run in tandem with work on comprehension. Use of alternative modes of communication to assist RV in communicating his message may be helpful. The communication folder suggested to supplement auditory comprehension could also be used by RV to achieve communication. Work in conjunction with his wife would be preferable so that she could maximise his use of alternative strategies in their interactions.

At the initial assessment, it was clear that RV and his wife had little understanding of his aphasia. Explanation with reinforcement through pictorial and written materials of the processing impairments underlying the difficulties that they are facing, and strategies that they can use to compensate for them, is likely to be valuable in developing and reinforcing more effective ways of coping and reducing anxiety. Such personalised materials are available in the ADA advice booklets (York Cognitive Neuropsychology Research Group, 1995) and the Glasgow Royal Infirmary computerised advice programme (Booth et al., 1999). As RV enjoys social clubs and also has a large family who live locally, he may also be able to use such booklets to educate other conversational partners. RV may also benefit from referral to the local stroke club. Besides providing him with a further social outlet, it would also give his wife some time for herself, which is important particularly given her high level of anxiety. Access to a carer support group, if available, may also be helpful for her.

Developing the hypotheses

> Remember that the results of assessment (and of intervention) feed back into developing the hypotheses you initially made. There may also be gaps in your interpretation, which the results have revealed. Use this page to write down what further investigations you might wish to consider to develop your hypotheses, some of which may depend on RV's response to therapy. As the assessments have focused mainly on understanding and speaking single words, you might wish at this stage to consider sentence processing and reading and writing deficits.

Our suggestions for developing the hypotheses

> Now read through the suggestions that we have made and compare them with your own.

The assessments undertaken leave a number of areas open for further exploration. While RV's performance on PALPA 48 *Written word–picture matching* fell within the range of the normal control subjects, it was below the mean. Furthermore, this assessment uses only items of high imageability. Further exploration of semantic processing abilites would be warranted in order to decide whether these contributed to RV's comprehension and word-finding deficits. This could initially be explored informally by examining ability to make semantic discriminations for items put into his communication folder. Further formal assessment could then be undertaken if the outcome of this indicated that it was warranted, e.g. through PALPA 50 *Written synonym judgements*, PALPA 51 *Word semantic association* or ADACB S1Wr *Synonym judgements*. These tasks would give information on whether abstract words reveal more impairment than high-imageability words.

The status of RV's phonological input lexicon could not be investigated because of his impaired phonological analysis. As he improves, it may become possible to test this, for example through use of PALPA 5 *Auditory lexical decision: imageability and frequency*.

Assessment has focused totally on single-word processing. Given the severe deficit that RV is experiencing functionally, it may be appropriate to explore his sentence processing abilities. The use of assessments that harnessed written input would allow central processing ability to be examined independently of the impact that his auditory processing deficits would have on sentence comprehension. Marshall, Black and Byng (1999) provide theory-based assessments which can be used to explore different underlying deficits in sentence comprehension.

It was suggested that RV and his wife may be encouraged to use alternative modes of communication to supplement his spoken output. Ability to use gesture could be examined, e.g. through use of the New England Pantomime Expression Test and Pantomime Referential Abilities Test (Duffy and Duffy, 1984). If this proves difficult, response to some preliminary training using a scheme such as Visual Action Therapy (Helm-Estabrooks, Fitzpatrick and

Barresi, 1982) could be illuminating. Drawing could also be explored (Lyon and Helm-Estabrooks, 1987; Lyon and Sims, 1989; Nicholas and Helm-Estabrooks, 1990). A conversation analysis would be helpful to investigate the current interactional strategies of RV and his wife (see Part Two).

Case 3
Mrs JA

When you work through this case remember to read the information first and then write down your own interpretation and ideas before you turn the page to read ours.

Initial impressions

> Read through the case description and think about what the important features are that will guide your selection of assessments.

Case description

JA is a 54-year-old housewife with three sons and two daughters from a first marriage. The children, now all grown up, live nearby. JA lives with her third husband; their relationship deteriorated, however, and she has expressed the intention of separating from him.

Before the stroke she had had three heart attacks, the stroke being precipitated by a fourth one. This resulted in a right hemiparesis and a severe aphasia, with receptive difficulties and expressive difficulties, which included effortful speech with oral struggling gestures. She received physiotherapy for her right hemiplegia for six weeks until she was discharged from hospital. JA's daughters reported that they think she has a hearing loss. They also commented that she had difficulty in recalling her children's names.

The speech and language therapist to whom she was referred assessed her at two months post onset on parts of the Boston Diagnostic Aphasia Examination (BDAE) with the following results.

1. On the auditory comprehension section, JA scored at the 50th percentile. On word discrimination, she correctly identified 6 out of 6 objects, 4 out of 6 actions, 3 out of 6 letters, 3 out of 6 colours, 2 out of 6 shapes, 5 out of 6

numbers and 10 out of 18 body parts. Eight of these correct responses took longer than 5 seconds. On the section that requires instructions to be followed, she correctly executed the commands with up to three components but omitted parts of the four and five part commands. She scored 1 out of 4 on the first four questions of the complex ideational material and became anxious when asked to do item five, which required her to answer questions on a short paragraph. Testing was therefore discontinued.

2. On the oral expression section, JA scored 6 out of 12 on non-verbal oral agility and 0 out of 12 on verbal oral agility. She scored 0 out of 10 on word repetition, with errors including inability to attempt a repetition, neologisms and phonemic paraphasias with apraxic distortions. She was not able to attempt phrase repetition. On word reading she scored 5 out of 30 on the Boston scoring system. The two items that she read correctly were the two monosyllabic items. For five out of the items she produced delayed phonemic paraphasias with evidence of articulatory searching. For one item she produced a neologism and did not attempt a further two out of the 10 items. On the responsive naming subsection she scored 12 out of 30 with two immediately correct responses, three delayed responses and five failures to produce a response. On visual confrontation naming, she scored 43 out of 105 on the Boston scoring system. For the 35 items, she produced correct responses for 12 and delayed correct responses for three. She produced eight semantic paraphasias (six of which were on the number section), three neologisms, four phonemic paraphasias and five failures to produce a response. All attempts had an apraxic quality.

A sample of her spontaneous speech at this time is given below, using a broad phonetic transcription which does not reflect her articulatory difficulties or oral struggles.

Sample of spontaneous speech

CP   who's waiting for you outside?

JA   oh Harry

CP   that your husband?

JA   yes I'll be (0.5) [mmmɛbɛ vɛɹi ɛdɛɪ] ah canna say er Harry seventy years on we've only been (1.0) one one work [beɪ]

CP   are you trying to say how long you've been married?

JA   I've only been er (1.0) I will be February

Sample of elicited speech (Cookie Theft Picture from the BDAE)

JA   the water there (.) that's like (3 syll.) down there (.) there boy (.) biscuit
biscuit (.) [feɪzɪŋ] off there (3.0).

CP   what's the girl doing?

JA   she wants something (.) fall off (2.0) I think he fallen there (1.0) bang.

A month later a further cerebrovascular accident was suspected affecting her right side; there was, however, no deterioration in her speech.

Your initial hypotheses

> Using the information given in the case description, consider the possible loci of JA's impairments. Given the limited information that you have, you may have several tentative hypotheses (the number of spaces provided is not intended as a guide). What is the justification for each of the hypotheses? What further information would you require to confirm or reject each of these?

If you want to keep the book unmarked, use the photocopiable sheets on pp. 232–239.

JA's difficulties compromise the

_____

Justification for this is that

_____

_____

_____

_____

_____

_____

_____

JA's difficulties compromise the

_____

Justification for this is that

_____

_____

_____

_____

_____

_____

JA's difficulties compromise the

_____

Justification for this is that

_____

_____

_____

_____

_____

JA's difficulties compromise the

_____

Justification for this is that

_____

_____

_____

_____

_____

_____

JA's difficulties compromise the

_____

Justification for this is that

_____

_____

_____

_____

_____

_____

What other factors need to be taken into consideration in planning assessments for JA?

Our hypotheses

> When you have completed your hypotheses, compare them to our suggestions. As you can see, it is not possible to propose firm hypotheses, but tentative possibilities can guide the selection of assessments, and each assessment should contribute to the identification of the level of deficit.

JA's difficulties compromise the allophonic realization system.

Justification for this is that JA is reported to have effortful speech with searching oral gestures, which may be associated with oral apraxia. Impaired performance on the non-verbal and verbal oral agility sections of the BDAE and the production of phonemic paraphasias, neologisms and phonetic distortions on the output tasks of repetition, naming and oral reading support the hypothesis of an impairment at this level.

JA's difficulties compromise the phonological assembly buffer.

Justification for this is that, although the phonetic distortions do strongly suggest an impairment in allophonic realisation, given the deficit that JA shows for all output tasks, it is not possible to rule out a concomitant impairment of the phonological assembly buffer.

JA's difficulties compromise the phonological output lexicon.

Justification for this is that even discounting articulatory difficulties, JA's performance on both responsive and visual confrontation naming is suggestive of a concomitant impairment at a higher level, with the production of semantic paraphasias, failures to respond and delayed responses. These error types could also be accounted for by impairment to the semantic system (see below).

JA's difficulties compromise the semantic system.

Justification for this is that she made errors on the word discrimination subtest, which has semantic distractors. A greater proportion of errors on the colours, letters and shapes items may indicate specific impairment to some semantic categories. The production of semantic paraphasias and failures to name on the visual confrontation subtest could also reflect a semantic impairment.

Other factors that need to be taken into consideration in planning assessment for JA include the hearing loss reported by JA's daughters, which may compromise her performance on assessments, the restricted use of her (dominant) right hand and the effect her limited communication may be having on her domestic situation.

Your selection of assessments

Now that you have some initial hypotheses about the loci of impairments, plan the types of assessment tasks that you would employ to test out your hypotheses. We have provided spaces for several assessments, but this does not mean that we expect you to use the exact number. You will find that selection of one assessment will be influenced by the potential findings of previous ones carried out.

Assessment
_____
_____

Justification for selection
_____
_____
_____
_____
_____
_____
_____

Assessment
_____

Justification for selection
_____
_____
_____
_____
_____
_____

Assessment
_____
_____

Justification for selection
_____

Assessment

Justification for selection

Assessment

Justification for selection

Assessment

Justification for selection

Our selection of assessments

> Now you have selected possible assessments compare them to the suggestions that we have made. Remember that there is no single right way of assessing someone using a psycholinguistic perspective. You should, however, be able to justify the need for each of the assessments in testing out specific hypotheses regarding the locus of impairment. If you selected different assessments, look at the assessments that were selected and work out the rationale behind this choice.

Assessment: Sections of the Apraxia Battery for Adults (Dabul, 1986).

Justification for selection: The Apraxia Battery will allow more detailed examination of the oral apraxia indicated by the BDAE results. It will also test whether she has a limb apraxia, which will be relevant if therapy is to be considered which uses gesture to supplement speech. Because the items in the Limb Apraxia subtest incorporate symbolic representations, such as 'indicating someone is crazy', this may also throw light on whether the conceptual use of symbols is retained. In respect of verbal problems the Apraxia Battery does not distinguish between ones which particularly compromise the phonological output buffer and those which compromise allophonic realisation; it does, however, provide clinically relevant information on whether errors increase or decrease on repeated attempts to say the same word, and on the effect of increasing word length.

Assessment: The recitation, singing and rhythm section of the BDAE.

Justification for selection: These sections of the BDAE will explore the extent to which 'overlearned' sequences in speech are retained, and may help to distinguish between difficulties in allophonic realisation (which would be reduced in overlearned sequences) and motor difficulties in articulation (which would not). The results could also indicate whether melodic line and rhythm could be used in therapy (as in Melodic Intonation Therapy; Sparks and Deck, 1985) to assist in overcoming her allophonic problems.

Assessment: The Mono-poly Naming Test, spoken and written.

Justification for selection: Performance on the spoken version of this naming assessment will provide information relevant to exploring the hypotheses made to explain JA's expressive difficulties. Comparison of JA's oral naming for mono-syllabic and polysyllabic items will provide information relevant to the status of the phonological assembly buffer and allophonic realisation. Examination of whether JA demonstrates a frequency effect will provide information relevant to the hypothesis that she has an impairment involving the phonological output lexicon. A comparison of her word retrieval abilities in oral and written input may also help to tease out whether JA has a central semantic impairment. If she shows a similar pattern of performance on both versions, this will either suggest a central deficit or that her written naming is mediated through the phonological output lexicon and the phonological assembly buffer. If she is able to retrieve words in written form which she is unable to retrieve orally, this will suggest that impaired semantic processing does not underlie impaired oral naming ability, and that direct access to the graphemic output lexicon from semantics is retained.

Assessment: Word–picture matching assessments in both spoken and written modalities. Possible assessments that could be used are PALPA 47 and 48 or ADACB S2 and S2Wr.

Justification for selection: These assessments will allow exploration of whether the auditory comprehension impairment identified on the BDAE and the semantic errors produced in oral naming arise as a consequence of impaired semantic processing. If this is the case, performance on both auditory and written modalities will be compromised. If performance is better on the written version, hearing or some aspect of auditory input processing may be impaired.

Assessment: Audiometric screening test.

Justification for selection: Given JA's relatives' reports of hearing difficulties, the audiometric screening test is essential in order to decide whether referral for a full examination is required. The findings of the hearing assessment will allow more objective consideration of the impact of hearing loss on JA's performance on assessments of auditory comprehension and on functional comprehension.

Assessment results

> Now read through the results of the assessments we carried out.

Apraxia Battery for Adults

JA obtained a perfect score on the Limb Apraxia subtest, indicating good use of her left hand for gesture and good retention of symbolic gesture. A score of 29 out of 50 confirmed that she has a significant degree of (non-verbal) oral apraxia, and evidenced several searching behaviours. She had a deterioration score of 0.6 on word repetition, as number of syllables increased from 1 to 3. On the Repeated Trials subtest she refused two items, and on six of the remaining eight items errors increased as she attempted to repeat the words. She showed 11 of the 15 features Dabul identifies as being characteristic of apraxia of speech.

The assessment also indicated that she had particular difficulty with words beginning with /v/, /r/, /l/ and /ʃ/, being more consistently accurate with plosives and nasals.

BDAE Recitation, singing and rhythm

JA was unable to recite the words for 'Happy Birthday' (used in preference to the nursery rhymes suggested in the test), or to hum the melody for this, and was unable to imitate tapping in rhythm beyond the first item.

Mono-poly Naming Test

A summary of JA's responses on the spoken version is given below, where a response is analysed as a phonemic paraphasia if an attempt contains 50% or more of the target phonemes and analysed as a neologism if it contains less than 50% of the target phonemes.

	Monosyllabic items	Polysyllabic items
Correct	4 out of 30 (13%)	0 out of 30 (0%)
Semantic/circumlocutions	2 out of 30 (7%)	4 out of 30 (13%)
No response	2 out of 30 (7%)	10 out of 30 (33%)
Phonemic paraphasias	11 out of 30 (37%)	6 out of 30 (20%)

| Neologisms | 8 out of 30 (27%) | 9 out of 30 (30%) |
| Spelling attempts | 3 out of 30 (10%) | 1 out of 30 (3%) |

In the responses scored as phonemic paraphasias and neologisms, JA frequently produced multiple attempts, for example:

'helicopter' → [ha hɔ mm hɛl pɔlɪbova pɔlɪɔtə]
'sphinx' → [kɹantzɪ kɹɔtə]

There were several examples of metathesis in JA's misproductions, e.g.[kunwən] for 'unicorn', some even in monosyllabic words e.g. [lei] for 'eel', [blɔt] for 'bolt'.

For the items where JA produced either a correct response or a phonemic paraphasia, 10 were of high frequency, six of medium frequency and six of low frequency.

The therapist provided phonemic cues for 35 items which were not named correctly. Following these, JA produced the correct item for three monosyllabic words, and six phonemic paraphasias (for two monosyllabic and four polysyllabic words).

In addition to the four responses that consisted solely of spelling out the target, JA also used this strategy in conjunction with phonological and neologistic errors. In all responses containing this strategy, she failed to spell out the word correctly. In only one instance did the use of spelling out appear to assist in getting a target related response:

'cigarette'   '   'c' 'r' 'i' 'g' 'a' 'r' 's' [sɪgaɹɛn]

There were frequent groping and searching behaviours, and prolongations of /s/ in JA's attempts. JA made comments that indicated that she knew the target and was aware that her attempts were not correct.

A written version of this test was given using a subset of 20 items, on which JA scored three correct. All were monosyllabic (fox (after self-correction), dart, bath). There were four refusals, all for polysyllabic words (kangaroo, cigarette, potato, umbrella). It was noted that she often attempted to spell out the word orally while writing, although these attempts were never correct. In the error items, she was almost consistently able to begin with the correct letter, and frequently showed knowledge of some later letters:

target	error
photographer	pho
grapes	grabes, *changed to* grapbes
screwdriver	swetdart
stork	swower, second attempt swo
helicopter	heth
match	mathes
dominoes	dir
muff	fleet
daffodil	deffowl
beak	benk, *changed to* baenk
elephant	e
mouse	mouch
harp	harch

PALPA 47 Spoken word–picture matching

JA made no errors on this assessment. Given her high level of performance, presentation of the written version of this assessment was not undertaken.

Audiometric screening test

Bilateral reduction of hearing by 30 dB and more was noted. It was particularly severe at high frequencies (70 dB and over in both ears).

Your interpretation of the results of the assessments

> What do the assessment results mean? Map out your hypotheses of the locus or loci of JA's comprehension deficit based on these findings, using the diagram of the model. Indicate also what processes seem to be preserved and which levels you are uncertain about from the assessment results so far. Note down the justification in support of your hypotheses.

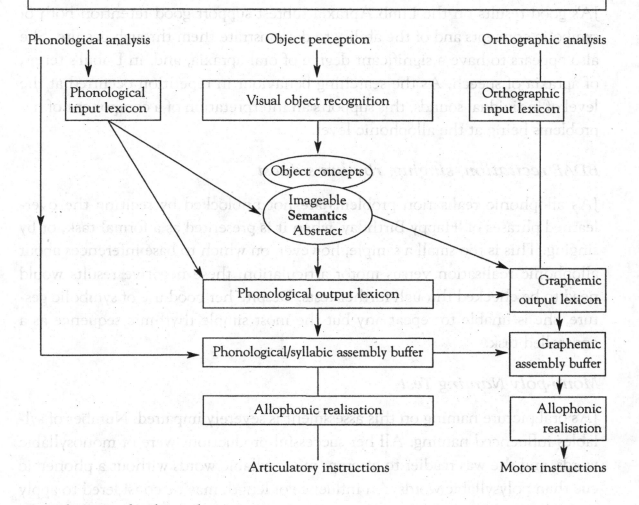

Justification for hypotheses

_____

_____

_____

_____

_____

_____

_____

Our interpretation of the results of the assessments

> Now read through our interpretation of the findings.

Apraxia Battery for Adults

JA's good results on the Limb Apraxia subtest support good retention both of symbolic concepts and of the ability to demonstrate them through gesture. She also appears to have a significant degree of oral apraxia, and, in Dabul's terms, of apraxia of speech. As the searching behaviour in repetition occurred at the level of individual sounds, this supports an interpretation of a component of her problems being at the allophonic level.

BDAE recitation, singing, rhythm subtest

JA's allophonic realisation problems are not unblocked by reciting the over-learned phrases of 'Happy Birthday' when it is presented as a formal task, or by singing. This is too small a sample, however, on which to base inferences about allophonic realisation versus motor articulation; these negative results would need to be checked through further tests. Despite her good use of symbolic gesture, she is unable to repeat any but the most simple rhythmic sequence as a controlled task.

Mono-poly Naming Test

JA's oral picture naming on this assessment is severely impaired. Number of syllables influenced naming. All her successful productions were of monosyllabic words, and she was readier to attempt monosyllabic words without a phonemic cue than polysyllabic words. An influence of length may be considered to apply at the level of the phonological assembly buffer, but it may also be a secondary effect due to the articulatory effort that has to be put into longer words. The number of metatheses suggests problems of seriation in the buffer, as well as of selection which may implicate both the buffer and allophonic realisation.

There was also a slight effect of frequency, with more correct items and phonemic paraphasias for high-frequency items, which may indicate that JA has an impairment in access to the phonological output lexicon. An impairment at this level could also explain the production of neologisms, although these may also be accounted for by severe impairment at the levels of phonological assembly and allophonic realisation.

JA produced a small number of semantic paraphasias and a larger number of failures to name. Both of these error types could be accounted for by a central semantic processing impairment. Her errorless performance on PALPA 47 *Spoken word–picture matching*, however, indicates intact semantic processing for at least high imageability items and therefore allows us to reject this hypothesis. These errors could be explained by impaired access to the phonological output lexicon. The greater number of no responses for polysyllabic items also suggests that impairments to the output buffer and allophonic realisation may also contribute to JA opting not to attempt a response. Provision of phonemic cues did not materially help her, and she frequently indicated that she knew what the intended word was but was unable to say it. This supports the interpretation that some of her difficulties lie in the realisation processes from the buffer output, i.e. allophonic shaping.

The rationale behind asking JA to undertake a written naming test was to allow comparison with spoken naming and, through this comparison, examine whether a central semantic impairment was present. As JA clearly demonstrated impairments to processes below the level of the semantic system, this makes the picture somewhat complex. Examination of her performance does, however, show that JA was generally able to access the word in the graphemic output lexicon, at least in part, since, with one exception, the words' initial letters were correctly accessed, and the vowel sound was generally correctly represented by the appropriate letter. This in turn provides further evidence to suggest that JA has intact semantic processing for high-imageability words. Her performance, with better performance for shorter words, is consistent with some impairment at the level of the graphemic assembly buffer. If the graphemic assembly buffer is influenced by the phonological assembly buffer (see Figure 4), this impairment in spelling may be secondary to JA's phonological difficulties. An alternative explanation could be of an independent functional lesion affecting the writing system.

JA spontaneously uses a strategy of spelling words orally when attempting spoken naming. Unfortunately this does not result in correct phonological realisations. Her selection of the initial letter under these circumstances seems to be inferior to that when the direct output is writing. This may indicate better direct access to the graphemic output lexicon from semantics than through the phonological output lexicon.

PALPA 47 Spoken word–picture matching

As noted above, JA's errorless performance on this assessment provides evidence for intact semantic processing for at least high-imageability words.

Audiometric screening test

The screening test confirms JA's daughters' view that she has a hearing loss.

Planning intervention

On the basis of the findings of the cognitive neuropsychological assessments it is proposed that JA's main difficulty in communicating lies at the allophonic level of speech production, although she has other subsidiary or secondary problems which implicate the phonological assembly buffer, the graphemic assembly buffer and the phonological output lexicon. She also has a degree of hearing impairment. What initial therapy would you derive from these findings?

Our suggestions for initial intervention

Now that you have thought about some possible interventions, compare them with our suggestions. Remember that these are only tentative ideas and may very well differ from yours. Both your and our ideas may be appropriate. The important issue is that intervention should be motivated by theoretical principles.

For direct work on JA's allophonic difficulties, a number of traditional programmes exist for therapy for apraxia of speech (Wertz, 1984). There is always an initial dilemma in employing these. Given the classical observation that automatic-reactive speech is better preserved than volitional-purposive speech (well demonstrated by JA during the Naming Test), the question is whether to use exercises that rely on meaningful whole words (which may be considered to be closer to the automatic), or whether to target the deficit head-on by practising meaningless combinations of sounds (although this relies heavily on the volitional). Wertz, LaPointe and Rosenbek (1984, p. 162) have suggested that there may be two types of apraxic talkers: those with more distortions than substitutions, who have an 'executive' apraxia, and those with more substitutions than distortions, who have a 'planning' apraxia. In psycholinguistic terms, the former may have greater impairment at the allophonic level and the latter at the level of the assembly buffer. Management of the two conditions may need to be different. For the second type, which seems to incorporate elements of a disorder of the phonological assembly buffer, remediation strategies such as segmentation and externalising representations through reading may be relevant. Wertz et al. advocate the use of meaningful items in treatment of both (putative) types, as being facilitative and motivating. They note, however, that some patients seem to have a dissociation of meaning and movement, so that meaning has no influence on their articulatory movements, or indeed may be inhibitory in that linguistic pressure moves too rapidly for the 'motor system' to respond in a coordinated fashion. In this case, practice with non-verbal movements and speech movements with and without voice may be the first approach in therapy.

As JA's naming problems are so severe (and, judging from the samples of speech provided, may be accompanied by possible problems in sentence construction, adding to the linguistic pressures on her), the initial suggestion for therapy for her allophonic difficulties may be to work on articulemes for phonetic placement of the articulators for the sounds with which she has consistent difficulties (Huskins, 1989; Square-Storer and Hayden, 1989). Due to her possible difficulties in hearing fricatives clearly, it may be preferable to concentrate on /l/ and /r/ rather than /v/ and /ʃ/. A possible complication may be her oral apraxia, although there is some evidence that oral and verbal apraxia may be dissociated (DeRenzi, Pieczuro and Vignolo, 1966). Although work with articulograms is intended to incorporate primarily kinaesthetic and visual feedback, it is frequently preceded by training in making auditory discriminations of the sounds to be worked on in articulation. In JA's case this would be difficult given her degree of hearing loss. The psycholinguistic model also does not propose an essential interdependence between auditory analysis and allophonic production. A multimodal approach, however, is often recommended in therapy, and in this case JA's good ability to read short single words could be used to reinforce the articuleme exercises.

To follow the work with articulemes, a programme using imitation of word contrasts, contrastive stress drills, reading cues, pairing gestures and speech, and use of a pacing board to organise speech production might be considered (see Chapter 10 of Wertz et al., 1984). LaPointe (1984) also describes treatment for case FB, using an evaluation design, and incorporating modeling by the clinician, with error explanation, word imitation, stimulation, demonstration, phonetic placement, repetition and expansion into phrases. Other traditional treatments for apraxia of speech are reviewed by Square-Storer (1989). One classical programme sometimes recommended for apraxia of speech, Melodic Intonation Therapy (Sparks and Deck, 1986) does not seem to be appropriate for JA, given her results on the recitation, melody and rhythm section of the BDAE.

All of the therapy approaches focused on remediating the impairment require a large amount of repetitive practice. It would therefore be important to establish whether JA has a family member or friend who could undertake regular practice with her. Given the tensions that exist between her and her husband, it is unlikely that JA will wish to undertake work with him.

The psycholinguistic analysis has shown that JA can reliably access through writing the first letter of a word she is trying to find, and that this access is easier through writing than through speech. She may therefore possibly be helped by having an alphabet board to hand on which she can indicate the first letter of the word she is struggling to find. Given the fairly limited success that phonemic cues had during the assessment of her picture naming, it is unlikely that she will be able to use the first letter information to cue her own production of a target item, but such information may be useful to her conversational partner in working out her target. This may be better at this stage than encouraging her spontaneous practice of sometimes spelling words aloud, as she appears to make more errors with this than when spelling in writing.

Symbolic gesture is another medium which seems to be relatively well preserved for her, although it would be desirable to confirm this finding by testing a wider range of items. (If these do present some difficulties, a formal training programme such as Visual Action Therapy (Helm-Estabrooks, Fitzpatrick and Barresi, 1982) could be considered.) All these communicative possibilities could be combined in a PACE programme (Promoting Aphasics Communicative Effectiveness; Davis and Wilcox, 1985).

In view of JA's deteriorating domestic relationships, with associated financial problems and her wish to move to separate accommodation from her husband, referral to social services and/or an advice centre for the disabled may be appropriate. Attendance at a Speech-after-Stroke Club may also provide her with alternative interests, company and sources of personal advice. Referral for a full audiometric assessment for consideration for a hearing aid should also be discussed with JA.

Developing the hypotheses

> Remember that the results of assessment (and of intervention) feed back into developing the hypotheses you initially made. There may also be gaps in your interpretation, which the results have revealed. Use this page to write down what further investigations you might wish to consider to develop your hypotheses, some of which may depend on JA's response to therapy.

Our suggestions for developing the hypotheses

> Now read through the suggestions that we have made and compare them with your own.

Testing JA's production difficulties by asking her to recite over-learned polysyllabic series like days of the week and months of the year may help to confirm that difficulties in allophonic realisation rather than articulation underlie her output. If she shows a superior ability to produce these sequences than sequences of unfamiliar polysyllabic words, this would support the hypothesis. It must be noted, however, that overlearned patterns could also reduce any assembly problems in the phonological assembly buffer.

As JA's allophonic difficulties become ameliorated, it may be possible to assess better the influence of phonological word assembly problems independently from these difficulties, through testing her ability to repeat non-words and shorter polysyllabic words (since the polysyllabic words included in the naming test were predominantly of three syllables).

Performance on the BDAE also highlighted comprehension deficits beyond the single word level. Assessment of sentence comprehension abilities could be undertaken to explore these, e.g. through PALPA 55 *Auditory sentence comprehension*. As no investigation of reading comprehension has been undertaken, it would be informative to examine this through PALPA 56 *Written sentence comprehension*, which would permit a direct comparison with auditory input.

The samples of speech in the case description also show some production difficulties at the sentence level, which should be analysed.

Assessment also identified impaired writing ability. If writing was important for JA, further assessment to pinpoint the nature of the writing impairment could be undertaken from which to develop intervention. Length and regularity could be explored systematically, to tease out influences attributable to the graphemic output buffer and the graphemic output lexicon, e.g. through PALPA 39 *Spelling to dictation: letter length* and PALPA 44 *Spelling to dictation: regularity*. Because of her hearing difficulties, it would be essential to check that JA could repeat correctly the dictated words. As JA spontaneously uses a strategy of oral spelling, her output in oral spelling and written spelling could be systematically compared, as it is known that these abilities can be dissociated (Lesser, 1990).

Part Two: Applying conversation analysis

Background

Conversation analysis (CA) differs from the majority of approaches that have been drawn upon to investigate aphasia in that it is not grounded in psychology or linguistics. Rather, CA has developed from the sociological practice of ethnomethodology. Pioneered by Garfinkel (1972), the focus of ethnomethodology is to understand how social order is achieved through the use of social methods adapted in a step-by-step procedure to the particular needs of any particular moment in interaction. From this perspective, social interaction is seen as an operation *achieved* by its participants rather than something static arising from internalised rules developed through socialisation.

Central to CA is a data-driven approach focused on what participants do rather than the imposition upon the data of the external analyst's categories, as in the cognitive neuropsychology (CN) approach. To understand the organisation of talk, CA examines how participants display to each other what is going on in the interaction. Evidence is sought inductively from the sequential unfolding of the interaction. Participants reveal directly, by their responses, their analysis of the preceding speaker's turn. A conversational turn is context-shaped in that it can only be understood with reference to the context from which it is built. It is also context-renewing in that it builds a context for what follows. The context is dynamic with utterances' meanings emerging from interactional work. This approach, therefore, emphasises the collaborative achievement of interaction with participants working together to negotiate meanings.

Using this empirical methodology, through detailed and repeated examination of naturally occurring conversation, conversation analysts have demonstrated talk's orderliness and explicated the details of conversational organisation, including the mechanisms of turn-taking, repair and topic management. Following an examination of the attractions of CA as a method of analysis for aphasic data, these areas will be reviewed and the consequences of aphasia for them discussed.

Conversation analysis and aphasia

Several features of CA make it a useful method to inform assessment and management of aphasia. First, the analysis is carried out on naturally occurring conversation. This contrasts with cognitive neuropsychological assessment which predominantly uses synthetic tasks (e.g. picture naming, word and non-word repetition). These are heavily abstracted from the interactional demands that the person with aphasia faces in his or her social context. Nevertheless there is an assumption that linguistic impairments and abilities identified in these tasks reflect those experienced on-line in interaction. Currently, however, there is very little information available on the relationship between performance on cognitive neuropsychological assessment and ability in conversation (although see Jones, 1984; Perkins, 1995a, b; Whitworth, 1995). In contrast, the use of conversational data provides high ecological validity because it provides analysis at the level at which intervention is ultimately targeted, i.e. maximising interactional ability. A further benefit of the use of everyday conversation is that it provides a minimally obtrusive assessment tool which reduces the stress that the person with aphasia may experience in undertaking formal assessments where the emphasis is on 'correct' performance. It is therefore a useful approach when working with people with aphasia who have a high level of anxiety in a testing situation.

CA's emphasis on the social role of language use provides an additional dimension to other approaches in aphasia assessment. As noted by Schiffrin (1988), language use involves more than the effective transmission and receipt of information. It is a 'vehicle through which selves, relationships and situations are socially constructed' (Schiffrin, 1988, p. 272). In aphasia, the compromised ability to engage in social life results, from a psychosocial perspective, in a handicap that is acutely experienced in virtually every aspect of daily living. Kagan and Gailey (1993) report that people with chronic aphasia attending the North York Aphasia Centre (in Canada) and their families cite loss of established relationships and social isolation as the major negative change in their lives. Within the family, the communication barrier created by aphasia frequently results in limiting interactions focused on specific physical needs or wants. There is a significant discrepancy between this type of interaction, often structured in a question–answer format, and the more flexible social conversation used in everyday life. CA's ability to identify such issues makes it a useful assessment method, highlighting issues which may be tackled in intervention.

Kagan (1995) further proposes that aphasia masks social and cognitive competence:

> When a person has difficulty in talking and understanding what is said, it is hard to see the active mind; it is difficult to envisage the capacity to make life decisions, and it is difficult to regard the person as a social being. These perceptions affect the way one is treated (p. 17).

She argues that the ability to engage in conversation is the key to revealing competence and being viewed as a social being, with important psychosocial benefits. The psychosocial benefits for people with aphasia of maintaining effective interaction to permit participation in social conversation are increasingly being recognised (Lyons, 1989; Kagan and Gailey, 1993).

A further advantage of a CA approach for aphasia is that it explicitly takes account of the minutiae of interaction, such as filled and unfilled pauses, repetitions and repairs (Lesser and Milroy, 1993). While such features are often ignored as 'messiness' in the data, they have interactional consequences which vary according to their sequential placement in the discourse. Furthermore, such minutiae are generally very common in aphasic conversation. For example, Perkins (1995a) demonstrates how, for one aphasic woman, the occurrence of long unfilled pauses within her conversational turns (which arose as a consequence of word-finding failures) led to her losing the conversational floor as her partner used the pauses to initiate a further turn. CA allows the precise description of the interactional consequences of particular linguistic impairments, providing a method to explore the consequences of impairments identified through cognitive neuropsychological assessment on interaction (Perkins, 1995a, b).

As discussed above, a central tenet of CA is that conversation is a collaborative achievement (Schegloff, 1982). As a consequence of this, successful aphasic interaction can be seen as the joint responsibility of both the impaired and non-impaired participants. This is demonstrated in the analysis of aphasic repair sequences by Milroy and Perkins (1992), which highlights the joint work of interlocutors collaborating to resolve trouble sources (see below for further discussion of repair organisation). While other work has acknowledged the need to examine the contribution made by the aphasic person's conversational partner(s) (e.g. Penn, 1985; Wirz et al., 1990), this is isolated and looked at as an independent phenomenon. CA's emphasis on conversation as a collaborative achievement, however, demonstrates that interaction is more than the sum of the contributions of the two halves; an essential component is the interlocutors' collaborative construction of the discourse. This has implications for both assessment and therapy, emphasising the need for coordinated work with the person with aphasia and partner together to develop successful interactional strategies.

CA provides principled procedures for judging success and failure based on sequential interactional outcome (i.e. how the conversational partner treats the preceding conversational turn). This avoids subjective judgements of appropriacy often used in functional communication assessments, which are necessarily based on some ill-defined notion of 'normality' (Lesser and Milroy, 1993). CA offers a framework that allows the characterisation of aphasic interaction without prior problematic assumptions of how this may relate to 'normal' interactional behaviour. While useful information can be gained from comparative analysis, the use of normal conversation as a benchmark for aphasic discourse is unsatisfactory. The person with aphasia does not have 'normal' interactional resources, but deviation from what is normal does not necessarily equate with failure or communicative ineffectiveness (Perkins, 1995a, b). As will be demonstrated below in the examination of repair organisation, the unique demands of aphasic discourse necessitate that it be treated autonomously if a clear insight is to be achieved into interactional management which can feed into the development of therapy.

In summary, CA is a data-driven approach, emphasising the description of observable behaviour and seeking evidence of interactional success or failure from the sequential context, i.e. the responses of the conversational partners. This offers a number of strengths to the aphasia therapist. Evidence is available in the data of (i) problems arising in conversation, (ii) strategies employed to deal with them and (iii) the outcome of the strategies. This information allows the therapist to develop interaction which is client-led and individually tailored to the unique interactional patterns that emerge from the linguistic impairments and strategies that have been developed by the person with aphasia and his or her key conversational partner. In the next section, three key aspects of conversational management, namely turn-taking, repair and topic management, are examined and the consequences of aphasia for their management discussed.

Conversational management and aphasia

Turn-taking

The organisation of turn-taking is fundamental to conversation. Turn-taking refers to the sharing of time and sequencing of contributions evident in any conversation, a turn being a conversational contribution by one speaker followed either by silence or by a contribution from another. In conversation, overwhelmingly one interlocutor speaks at a time with frequent split second transition from one speaker to the next. Sacks, Schegloff and Jefferson (1974) propose that the mechanism which accounts for this split-second timing is a set of rules which operates on a turn by turn basis as a sharing device for the right to take the conversational floor. They propose that turns are made up of *turn constructional units* determined by syntactic and prosodic features. Speakers may change at the end of a turn constructional unit, which is known as a *transition relevance place*. It is the projectability of the end of turn constructional units which accounts for the common occurrence of split second speaker transition. As illustrated in *(i)* below, however, turns often consist of more than one turn constructional unit (# marks the end of turn constructional units).

(i)

A   I says why# and then I got something for the dole for the council offices# I take that up and all# I says there you are# fill that in I says and I'll tell you all you want to know#

Given that overlapping speech is relatively infrequent, it is necessary to ask how speakers distinguish between non-final and turn-final turn constructional units. A range of research has identified phonetic, prosodic and non-verbal phenomena which appear to have important roles in indicating turn completion (Local, Kelly and Wells, 1986; Local, 1986; Duncan, 1972; Ellis and Beattie, 1986).

Speaker transition can be achieved by the current speaker selecting the next speaker by, for example, asking a question or selecting him or her by name. Where a speaker does this, speaker transition should occur at the next transition relevance place. Where the next speaker is not selected, any speaker may self-select at a transition relevance place, the first speaker gaining rights to the next turn. This includes the current speaker taking a further turn constructional unit and continuing with his or her turn, as well as another speaker self-selecting and effecting speaker transition.

On the basis of these turn-taking rules, silence may have different interactional consequences. Where there has not been explicit next speaker selection, a silence after a transition relevance place represents a lapse in conversation, as seen after T(urn) 3 of the following excerpt from a conversation between a man with aphasia and his brother [see also extract *(xix)*]. (As in all the extracts we use, the person with aphasia is identified as AP, and the conversational partner as CP.)

(ii)
1.   CP   do you want half a pie?
2.   AP   no thanks no I'm not ready for it no not ready for anything yet
3.   CP   you can have half a pie
          (5.0)
4.   AP   I want to see what she knows about this thing going right now

This contrasts to a silence after a transition relevance place when there has been selection of the next speaker. This represents an *attributable silence* in which the silence can be attributed to the person who has been selected but who has not produced his or her turn. The following extract is taken from a conversation between two unimpaired individuals:

(iii)
A   is there something bothering you or not?
     (1.0)
A   yes or no
     (1.5)
A   eh?
B   no
(Atkinson and Drew, 1979: p. 52)

In this extract, A asks B a question, thus selecting B as next speaker. The following 1-second silence can be analysed as attributable to B, who has not produced his turn. A's orientation to B's silence (and withholding of his turn) is demonstrated by the question being repeated, providing clear evidence of speaker expectations.

Given the multiplicity of cues which are available for transition relevance places (syntactic, prosodic, non-verbal), it is unlikely that auditory comprehension difficulties as such would materially influence turn-taking in most aphasic people. Excessively long turns, however, have been reported in fluent aphasia with impaired ability to self-monitor (Edwards and Garman, 1989). In contrast, production difficulties may have a significant impact. Because of the split-second timing which turn-taking requires, linguistic deficits may compromise the ability of the person with aphasia to secure the conversational floor or to hold onto it. Particularly in multi-party conversations, where there is more competition for the conversational floor, the person with aphasia may have difficulty producing a turn quickly enough at a transition relevance place to secure a right to the floor. The impact of this will be to impede his or her ability to initiate in the conversation, thus resulting in a passive role with contributions only possible when explicitly given the floor by the current speaker asking a question.

Even when people with aphasia are explicitly given the conversational floor, if their linguistic impairments preclude them from being able to produce a turn quickly, this may have a number of interactional consequences. Under the pressure of the normal turn-taking rules which, as discussed above, result in silences after questions being treated as attributable and accountable, the person with aphasia may attempt to produce his or her turn quickly. This can give rise to numerous linguistic errors which may need repair work to resolve before he or she can complete the turn. Alternatively, the person with aphasia may delay in responding, giving him or herself extra processing time to formulate the turn. The interactional consequences of this will depend on how the conversational partner responds to the resulting attributable silence. In the following extract, the conversational partner selects his wife, who is aphasic, as the next speaker through the use of a question.

(iv)

1. CP   is there anything you [f] you fancy having in for your (1.3) meals for
         next week?
         (6.0)
2. AP   [wə] well when especially when when you're off erm (6.2) we can [aʔ]
         well (2.5) have something (3.2) a little bits [s] little bits of (2.3) nice
         things
3. CP   at lunch time?

The 6-second silence which is attributable to AP is not treated as a problem in the interaction as was seen in *(ii)* above. The silence is tolerated and after it AP produces her turn. The analysis carried out on the conversation between this couple showed that a high tolerance of silences was a feature of their interaction, a strategy which may have developed to cope with the impact of AP's language impairment on interaction. This can be seen as a joint strategy; while CP can be seen to be tolerating these silences, AP is actually 'producing' them by delaying the start of her turn. As it is a joint strategy, AP may experience different interactional outcomes to her 'production' of long silences with different conversational partners who have not developed tolerance of them. This may be an issue worth exploring in therapy.

Extract (iv) also demonstrates that AP produces long silences within her conversational turns, a common feature of aphasic discourse. CP is also tolerant of silences within turns and this appears to be beneficial to the interaction as AP is able to complete her turn when given the time to do so. Silences in this position can, however, make the person with aphasia vulnerable to loss of the floor if the silence is used by the conversational partner to gain a turn at talk. This is seen in the following extract with another pair of speakers.

(v)
1.   AP   yes I've got a er a I've got a lot on there now I've got I've got (1.0)
2.   CP   have you been talking up home?

The person with aphasia produces a 1-second unfilled pause within his turn, which from the syntactic shape is clearly not complete. CP uses the silence to take the conversational floor and initiate a new topic without allowing AP to complete his TI contribution. If this happens frequently, the person with aphasia may be unable to influence the topic of conversation as his or her attempts to contribute are continuously glossed over. People with aphasia may be able to exploit non-verbal cues to indicate that they have not completed their turn. Ahlsen (1985) reported that a raised hand was used by some of the aphasic participants as a turn-holding signal to avert loss of the floor, the hand being dropped to signify completion. Conway (1990) also described one woman with aphasia who altered her body posture, sitting forward to signal that her turn was still in progress and relaxing this position when she had finished her turn at talk.

Tokens such as 'mm', 'aha', 'yeah', 'right' pervade conversation and have been the focus of much attention in both the linguistic and CA literature. While such tokens have frequently been treated as an aggregate, Schegloff (1982) criticises this approach, arguing for the need to examine their function in their sequential environment. Such tokens, when they occur in isolation (which we will refer to as minimal turns), function to waive the opportunity to take a fuller turn at talk and pass the floor back to the conversational partner.

By foregoing the chance to take a fuller turn, the speaker is passing the opportunity to initiate repair, leading to the inference that the previous turn is understood. Such tokens can therefore be seen to express a claim of understanding. Schegloff also describes their continuer usage in which the speaker, by producing such a token, demonstrates understanding that an extended unit of talk is underway by another and that it is not yet complete. Jefferson (1984) also describes the use of these tokens in certain sequential contexts to avoid taking the conversational floor, which she calls *passive recipiency*. She provides data to illustrate that passive recipiency can be used to avoid movement into speakership even where it is appropriate leading to the *perverse passive*. Extract *(vi)* below from Jefferson (1984: p. 209) illustrates this phenomenon in unimpaired speakers (Jefferson's transcription conventions are used):

(vi)

```
40.   G    'hhhhhh I'm not going to uhm, hh maybe queer a dea:l just by want-
            ing this that and the other (you know)
41.                                         [
42.   B                                     NO::
43.        (0.2)
44.   G    'hhhh s:So: uhm,h (.) tha:t's the story.
45.   B    Mm hm,
46.        (0.2)
47.   G    An:d uh (0.6) uhm,hhh (1.0) 'hhhh u-Then I have a ma:n coming
            Tue:sday to see abou:t uh remo:deling the kitchen the way I want it
            you know? and the butler's pa:ntry
```

An example of the perverse passive can be seen in T45. In her previous turn, G has marked the completion of the telling with 'that's the story'. This is an appropriate place for B to take a full turn. Instead, she produces 'mm hm', which results in G taking another turn. The self-repair suggests that G was perhaps not expecting the floor to be returned back to her so quickly.

Lesser and Milroy (1993: pp. 220ff) comment that in view of these tokens' interactional function, limited linguistic substance and lack of semantic content, it is not surprising that aphasic speakers make extensive use of them. Given the impact of the variety of possible linguistic deficits on an aphasic speaker's ability to produce a full turn at talk, the use of minimal turns allows interactive participation in a conversation while effectively placing the onus of the conversation on the conversational partner. In a pilot study examining videos of conversations between pairs of people with Broca's aphasia, Fleming (1989) found that the weaker participant in each dyad used a large number of minimal turns, which appeared to have the function of passive recipiency proposed by Jefferson (1984). By producing these tokens, the participants were able to take an active role in the conversation while minimising the need to produce conversational turns which would make a greater demand on his or her limited linguistic resources. Perkins (1995a) describes a similar phenomenon in a conversation between an aphasic woman and her relative with the use of minimal turns being used to avoid taking full turns at talk, which may reveal linguistic incompetence as illustrated in (vii) below (minimal turns are marked with *):

(vii)
1.	CP	yeah so (3.5) looking forward to tonight eh?
		(1.5)
*2.	AP	yes
3.	CP	should be interesting
		(3.0)
*4.	AP	erm well yes
5.	CP	{hehehheheh}
*6.	AP	{heheheh} <yes>
7.	CP	<well> we'll see how see how she can do with a vegetarian menu eh?
*8.	AP	yes
9.	CP	{heheheh}
*10.	AP	{eheheheheh}
		(1.5)
*11.	AP	<mm>
12.	CP	<(2 syll.)> if that was all she could think of
		(3.5)
13.	CP	eh?
		(2.0)
14.	AP	alright (5 syll.)

In this extract AP resists movement into speakership by producing minimal turns which pass the conversational floor back to CP and impose responsibility for maintenance of the conversation on him.

Different turn-taking management issues arise in interaction with people with fluent aphasia who have poor ability to monitor. People with these types of deficit do not have difficulty securing the conversational floor to take major turns. Rather, they have a tendency to exploit the mechanisms of turn taking and fail to hand over the conversational floor. Edwards and Garman (1989) describe the discourse of a fluent aphasic patient who produced excessively long and semantically opaque turns at talk. They suggest that this 'press of speech' may arise from not being able to satisfy the lexical demands of the message level in a sufficiently precise way because of a lexical retrieval deficit. They propose that he is carrying to an extreme a pattern of behaviour characteristic of normal speakers. When they experience temporary word-finding difficulties, they also tend to run on until interrupted. An example of this type of behaviour is seen in (viii) below:

(viii)

1. AP   it looks after you I've got to be careful I go every of every m- well it used to be before one two weeks now I can just they can get hold of me with er at the moment a month and have a look at you and have a look at your blood have a look at it and see what it is and of course you've got to have all your things and you got to they start off nice all the things you get *(shows medical card)* that's alright that's terrible they get panicky.
2. CP   is this your blood pressure?
3. AP   no its erm its well well I never it's warfarin.
4. CP   ah yes

The person with aphasia takes a protracted turn consisting of many turn constructional units. Overall the turn is lexically empty but the fast rate of speech he uses makes it difficult for the conversational partner to get the conversational floor to initiate repair. The strategy employed by the conversational partner (T2) is to eventually initiate repair based on a concrete referent which is supplied (the medical card). This demonstrates that she has misunderstood what the previous turn was about (warfarin not blood pressure).

Repair

As we have already discussed, conversation is sequential, with each turn being built in relation to the prior turn. However, a variety of trouble sources can arise in interaction, which provides an obstacle to the production of a sequentially implicated next turn. Examples of trouble sources include the need to change the message, false starts, dysfluencies, mishearings and misunderstandings. Conversation analysts use the term *trouble source* in preference to error, since there is no one-to-one relationship between the two. Speakers may revise their utterances when there is no identifiable error and conversely may ignore error or ambiguity if it does not impede the ability to produce a sequentially relevant next turn. This is an important point for aphasia, because it suggests that not all aphasic errors will necessarily be trouble sources requiring repair work. The organisation of repair provides a mechanism to deal with trouble sources. Repair organisation is a particularly important device for the communication disordered population given the variety of potential trouble sources which may impede the progression of conversation (Milroy and Perkins, 1992).

In their examination of repair, Schegloff, Jefferson and Sacks (1977) make two important distinctions: first, *self-initiated* versus *other-initiated* repair, which refers to repair by a speaker respectively with or without prompting; second, *self-repair* carried out by the speaker versus *other-repair* carried out by another participant. Repairs are organised according to the participants' opportunities to carry them out, leading to a preference for self-repair over other-repair and a preference for self-initiation over other-initiation of repair. The modulation of other-repair into a question format is a common feature. Schegloff et al. suggest that the reason for this is that, when hearing or understanding is adequate for the production of correction by other, it is adequate for the production of a sequentially relevant next turn. This accounts for the paucity of other-repair; those who could do them do a sequentially relevant next turn instead. Other-repair, when it does occur, is frequently reacted to as socially sensitive. This issue will be discussed further below.

A number of key questions can be asked in assessment of the repair abilities of people with aphasia and their conversational partners. For a person with an impairment which compromises comprehension, it may be important to ask whether he or she can initiate repair on the conversational partner's turn (other-initiated repair), i.e. request that the conversational partner clarifies all or part of his or her earlier turn. Ability to do this may be an important strategy to enhance the level of comprehension in conversation. Absence of other-initiated repair by the person with impaired comprehension may arise for a number of different reasons. First, it may be that despite deficits identified from cognitive neuropsychological assessment, in an interactional setting this does not impede comprehension. Second, a person with aphasia may choose not to initiate repair because he or she does not want to reveal failure in comprehension. Finally, he or she may not be aware of misunderstanding.

Another key question in the examination of repair abilities is whether the person with aphasia is able to initiate repair on his or her own turn (self-initiation), i.e. show awareness of potential trouble sources. Frequently, this is a retained ability although the person with aphasia, having recognised a trouble source, may not then have the linguistic resources to self-repair as seen in the following extract:

(xiii)

1. AP   and once I get those done I'll have to cut all the er trousers the the the
2. CP   the trees
3. AP   the trees that's right

AP initiates repair on a lexical mis-selection by starting a replacement of the noun phrase with repetition of 'the'. He does not, however, effect self-repair before CP carries out other-repair by providing 'the trees'.

For people who have poor self-monitoring ability, however, self-initiation of repair may be problematic and this will have interactional consequences as illustrated in the following extract:

(xiv)

1.   AP   [tʃɪpsɛɪ sɛt] what does Walter to do with them?
2.   CP   eh?
3.   AP   what's he gonna do what's he gonna
4.   CP   he's coming in about an hour he's pubbing isn't he?
5.   AP   he's what?
6.   CP   he's coming to pick you up in about an hour
7.   AP   who's back by what's that for?
8.   CP   Douglas
9.   AP   oh he's coming is he ah
10. CP   he's coming down here
11. AP   ah

AP produces a turn with a neologism, a semantic paraphasia on the name 'Walter' (as Walter is the CP that he is talking to, it is likely that he is referring to another family member) and a deictic referring expression 'them', which has no traceable antecedent in the conversation. AP does not, however, self-initiate repair work, indicating lack of awareness that the turn contains potential trouble sources. CP other-initiates repair with 'eh?', which AP deals with by redoing the problematic turn referring to the male referent as 'he'. CP produces a sequentially relevant next turn (T4) which reveals that his understanding that the original semantic paraphasia 'Walter' in T1 and 'he' in T3 refers to AP's son. The repair sequence that follows, however, in particular AP's other-initiation of repair on the referent that CP is talking about in T7 ('who') suggests that CP has misunderstood to whom AP was originally referring in T1 and T3. This extract demonstrates well how repair work halts the current interactional business as it becomes the interactional business in its own right. The repair work overrides the topic from AP's question in T1 and it is abandoned.

In normal interaction, repair organisation deals rapidly with trouble sources. It is overwhelmingly carried out within the turn in which the trouble source appears (self-initiated self-repair), with less preferred forms of repair (other-initiated and other-repair) overwhelmingly being resolved within two further turns (although see Schegloff, 1987, 1992, on third and fourth position repairs). In aphasic interaction, however, rapid repair work is often not achieved, giving rise to different interactional issues for the interlocutors to negotiate. Milroy and Perkins (1992) propose that repair in aphasic discourse often has a complex organisation, which appears to be structurally different in several aspects from repair organisation in normal discourse. For the person with aphasia, linguistic impairments give rise to the need for greater use of repair work. The same linguistic impairments may, however, limit his or her ability to execute self-repair within the turn of the trouble source. As a consequence, the fast resolution of repair seen in normal conversation is often not accomplished and successful repair outcomes can be described as collaboratively achieved rather than completed by 'self' or 'other'.

Milroy and Perkins propose that Clark and Schaefer's (1987, 1989) CA-motivated model of conversational contributions provides a useful framework to capture the complexity of aphasic repair organisation. The model stresses the collaborative nature of conversation, with contributions to conversation having two constituents: the *presentation phase*, where an utterance is presented by the contributor (interlocutor A); and the *acceptance phase*, which is initiated by the listener (interlocutor B) but which involves both interlocutors working to establish that B has reached an understanding of A's presentation sufficient for current purposes. This phase may constitute either positive evidence of understanding (in the form of acknowledgement tokens or moving on to the next relevant contribution) or initiation of repair work.

Central to the model is *the principle of least collaborative effort*, whereby participants strive to minimise the total effort spent on a contribution in both the presentation and acceptance phases. There is generally a trade-off in effort between initiating a presentation and refashioning it, in that the greater the effort expended on designing a presentation, the less is needed for acceptance. This accounts for the preference for self-repair, in which effort is expended to design a presentation which can achieve immediate acceptance. A number of factors may, however, give rise to presentations which require collaborative repair work to achieve completion of the acceptance phase. Milroy and Perkins suggest that the principle of least collaborative effort can be seen to be operating in aphasic conversations, in that less overall collaborative effort is required if the unimpaired conversational partner contributes to the repair work to achieve acceptance of a presentation than if the aphasic partner works in isolation to try and design an immediately acceptable presentation (a task which may be beyond his or her linguistic abilities). Collaborative sequences, which may persist over a large number of turns are, therefore, a common phenomenon of aphasic interaction. Analysis of the manner in which the person with aphasia and his or her conversational partner work together to resolve trouble sources can be an extremely valuable part of assessment. Extract *(xv)* is a collaborative repair sequence from a conversation between a woman with aphasia and her husband:

(xv)
1. AP   anyway I'll tell you where we supposed to be going erm (1.0) in a few weeks er from (7.0) erm what do they call it [wə] (2.0)
2. CP   work
3. AP   no from the Tuesday
4. CP   g<roup>
5. AP   <[wə]> aha what do they call it?
6. CP   er [faʊn faʊ<n>]
7. AP   <the> [faʊn] Fountain (1.2) the Fountain (3.0) ee I don't know I'm very I'm not very sure
8. CP   okay well where are you going what are you
9. AP   we're going to (4.2) the (4.0) [ ] no (2.8) the (4.2) hhhh in it's in (1.5)
         what do they call it erm in Whickham

10. CP Whickham?
11. AP Whickham (1.5) the (2.3) [kə] the (2.6)
12. CP the baths
13. AP no no no {hehehehhe} the [grɛɪ] not the <[grɛɪ]>
14. CP <the> garden centre?
15. AP yes
16. CP the garden centre
17. AP aha well it's it's the (1.5)
18. CP council
19. AP aha
20. CP so it's the council garden cen<tre>
21. AP <the[kaʊn]> council (1.4)
22. CP garden centre
23. AP garden <centre>
24. CP <centre> fine
25. AP and we're going to have a look around there
26. CP oh that's good

In AP's T1 there is evidence of problems in lexical retrieval with a 7-second unfilled pause followed by filled delay and comments. She finally produces '[wə]' followed by a 2-second unfilled pause after which CP initiates collaborative work by putting forward a possible candidate for completion based on the partial phonological attempt. AP, however, rejects this in T3 and then goes on to provide information ('from the Tuesday'), which CP uses to propose an alternative candidate for understanding in T4. While AP accepts this, this is not the end of the collaborative repair sequence as AP pursues the establishment of the exact name of the group. Collaborative work continues around this issue until T7, when AP aborts the search with 'ee I don't know I'm not very sure'. CP accepts this, the original trouble source is negotiated and the conversation then moves on as marked by CP's question in T8. This sequence demonstrates that the understanding sufficient for current purposes to allow the conversation to proceed is not fixed but is negotiable, requiring collaborative work.

AP again runs into word-finding difficulties in T9 and collaborative work to establish where they are going continues until T25, when the conversation moves from resolution of the trouble source to develop the topic further. In both of the collaborative repair sequences in this extract, the importance of the two participants working together to achieve repair is demonstrated. While AP is not able to quickly effect self-repair and is assisted by the activity of her conversational partner, she is not taking a passive role. The information that she provides (for example, the circumlocutory information in T3 and T9, the phonological information in T13 and the requests for and attempts at further information in T5 and T17) contributes to a quicker resolution than that which would have been achieved if she had simply continued to search, leaving CP to attempt to collaborate with very little information on which to base his attempts.

Analysis has shown that conversationalists are socially sensitive in their orientation to repair work. If the problem necessitating repair can be traced back to some personal insufficiency, it becomes an event which threatens face (Goffman, 1955; Couper-Kuhlen, 1992). Jefferson (1987) demonstrates that a characteristic of other-repair is an accounting for lapses in conduct which have given rise to repair work. Such accounting is a common feature of aphasic repair (Perkins, in press), as seen in (xvi) which occurs at the end of a protracted collaborative repair sequence in which the person with aphasia and her conversational partner have been dealing with a word retrieval failure for the name of a local hospital (Prudhoe):

(xvi)
1. CP Prudhoe
2. AP thank you
3. CP right
4. AP I now I cannot get that out do you know that is one of the things I
        cannot get it out

Wilkinson (1995) has addressed the social sensitivity of repair in aphasic conversation. In relation to Sack's (1984) proposal that deviations from 'being ordinary' are accountable and require interactional work to avoid potentially negative interactional incidents, Wilkinson proposes that displays of non-competence in aphasia are interactionally delicate, bringing to the conversational surface the issue of the person with aphasia being a 'non-ordinary' interactant. He identifies a sequential pattern around trouble sources in conversations between therapists and patients. The patient laughs and often makes some form of account for the lapse in competence. In the next turn the therapist resists affiliating with the laughter and does not comment verbally on the lapse. Parallels can be drawn between this pattern and that seen in talk about troubles

(Jefferson, 1984), in which the troubles-teller uses laughter as a resource to display that he or she is coping with the trouble. Since laughter can be viewed as treating the trouble lightly, the troubles-recipient does not affiliate with the laughter but instead exhibits concern about the trouble. Wilkinson suggests that the therapist, by withholding laughter, is attempting to keep the non-ordinary identity off the conversational surface.

An interesting issue which arises from the sensitivity of repair is the impact of pursuing correction of aphasic errors even where this is unnecessary for understanding. As highlighted in extract (xv) above, the resolution of a trouble source is not fixed but is negotiable. The following extract between a woman with aphasia and her husband shows that repair may be extended beyond establishing mutual understanding to achieve correct production by the person with aphasia.

(xvii)
1.   AP   and I'll tell you what I want I need some (2.5) o::h (2.5) it's it's a [də] 'd'
2.   CP   [də]?
3.   AP   a (2.4)
4.   CP   to eat?
5.   AP   no it's a (3.0) it's not a 'd' a [dɪ]a death no
6.   CP   a death you don't want a death
7.   AP   {laughter} shush I'm thinking it's a (2.0) death no {heh}
8.   CP   er (1.0)
9.   AP   [dɛʃ]
10. CP   dish?
11. AP   dish thank you dish (1.5)
12. CP   washer
13. AP   wipe wipe
14. CP   a dish wipe
15. AP   wiper aha
16. CP   a dish cloth
17. AP   mhm
18. CP   a what?
19. AP   er what?
20. CP   dish cloth
21. AP   dish (1.0)
22. CP   cloth

23. AP   cloth cloth
24. CP   a dish cloth
25. AP   dish cloth
26. CP   fine
27. AP   erm because Steven (1.5) I don't know what he's done with those ones that I've got but they're (1.5) they're terrible

AP initiates repair in T1 as she attempts to deal with the failure in lexical retrieval. She provides some phonological and orthographic information. CP uses this to initiate collaborative repair, picking up on the phonological cues given by AP as well as giving feedback about phonological errors (T6). He also tries to gain some semantic information about the target (T4). AP rejects the suggestion and then goes back to lexical searching. By T16 CP has provided a candidate understanding which AP conforms with 'mhm' in T17. CP does not, however, permit the repair sequence to be closed down but pursues a correct production of 'dish cloth' by providing various models for repetition before the repair sequence is closed down and the conversation continues in T27. CP's pursuit of a correct production from AP extends the time out from the main interactional business and keeps AP's aphasic identity (and linguistic incompetence) on the conversational surface.

Given the sensitivity of protracted repair in exposing failures in competence, an option open to interlocutors is to opt for a non-repair way of dealing with a potential trouble source by passing over it altogether (Heritage and Atkinson, 1984). This option is open to both the person with aphasia (as discussed above in relation to comprehension impairments) and to the conversational partner. While for some people with aphasia, the occasional glossing over of a potential trouble source may not have great consequences, Perkins (in press) presents data on one case which highlights that her partner's strategy of not initiating repair on her turns severely limits her ability to actively contribute to the interaction. As she does not successfully make a contribution to conversation, she is unable to influence the development of the topic and as a consequence is forced into a passive role, as is seen in the following extract:

(xviii)
1. CP   Letts Way but I don't know what er three weeks since I was talking to her and she said well [wə] I'll be away shortly
2. AP   aha

3.	CP	but I don't know whether \<she was with her>
4.	AP	\<no(2 syll. just)> she was er (1.2) daughter was waiting for some t‑
5.	CP	'cause she's got a house
6.	AP	oh
7.	CP	down there 'cause he's in the police thing down there now in the in \<the> gaol
8.	AP	\<aah>
7cont.CP		he's got his job er he's off the buses now he's in the on\<the> on the gaols thing
9.	AP	\<ah>
7cont.CP		now you see and I thought the way she was talking I thought she might have been away about a fortnight
10.	AP	no she was [wə] she was supposed to er (0.6) I've forgotten but she was but she was (1.6)
11.	CP	I was talking to her at the butchers down down the bottom and she \<was> telling us she says oh I'll not be long before I'm going
12.	AP	\<mm> (1.2)
13.	AP	\<mm>
14.	CP	\<I> says you ganning for good or what she says I'm not sure it's it's a big house she's I'm going to live with them
15.	AP	aye but er but she (1.8) eee I don't know what she said
16.	CP	that's what she said to me anyway hinny and I thought maybe you'd heard it whether she'd moved or not you \<see>
17.	AP	\<no>

In T4, T10 and T15, AP attempts to make a contribution to the conversation but runs into difficulty. CP does not, however, initiate collaborative repair but continues to develop the topic without AP's turns contributing further to the conversation.

Topic management

Topic can loosely be defined as 'what is talked about through some series of turns at talk' (Lesser and Milroy, 1993, p. 204). Topical coherence can be seen to be something that is constructed across turns by the collaboration of participants. As reported by Sacks (1992), there is a preference for topics to be related to prior ones. Conversationalists can be seen to work to achieve stepwise topic relatedness in which one topic flows into another. Boundaried topical movement, in which closure of one topic is followed by initiation of another, can be seen to be marked in a number of ways as conversationalists orient others to the new topic. One way in which this is done is through the use of misplacement and discontinuity markers such as 'by the way', 'hey' (Schegloff, 1979). Button and Casey (1984) describe the use of topic initial elicitors to invite new topics from conversational partners. Fasold (1990) has suggested that the sequential organisation of topic is, in effect, a by-product of the turn-taking system which favours the production of utterances with minimum gap or overlap. If a gap does occur which is not attributable to any participant, speakers may assume that nobody has anything further to say about what is currently being discussed and introduce a new topic. The use of a gap as a topic boundary is a common feature in conversation.

Initiation of a new topic can be problematic for the person with aphasia, since if he or she runs into difficulties with a turn, it may be more difficult to carry out collaborative repair than to attempt repair where the topic is already established thus providing a framework of shared knowledge. As has already been discussed in relation to extract (xviii) above, if the conversational partner chooses to opt for a strategy of glossing over problematic turns, rather than risking initiating or extending collaborative repair work, this can force people with aphasia into a passive role in the conversation, in which they respond rather than initiate. Extract (xix) below is taken from a conversation between a man with aphasia and his brother.

(xix)
1. CP do you want half a pie?
2. AP no thanks no I'm not ready for it no not ready for anything yet
3. CP you can have half a pie
   (5.0)
4. AP I want to see what she knows about this thing going right now
5. CP eh?
6. AP what she [seɪfni] what she [seɪf] do you think or not what she saying what she saying?
7. CP I don't know {hahaha}
8. AP {heh}

After a 5-second lapse in the conversation, AP initiates a new topic in T4. Evidence for failure to orient his conversational partner to the new topic is provided by CP's general repair initiator in T5. CP first requests clarification (T5), to which AP attempts a repair. This is not, however, successful and the conversational partner is then seen in T7 to close down the topic with 'I don't know' and laughter. The outcome of this is that the new topic is not developed in the conversation.

This extract highlights that maintenance of topics can also be problematic in aphasia. The following extract is from a conversation from the same speakers as in (*xix*).

(*xx*)
1. AP   mm not so bad hhh I've got one I gonna gonna (1 syll.) tonight I've got to go and er go [naɪə] tomorrow
2. CP   go up where?
3. AP   (1 syll.)
4. CP   stroke centre?
5. AP   I'm going a I'm going out tomorrow not ['sərɛ'nɛɪkə]
6. CP   stroke centre?
7. AP   yes yeah
8. CP   I thought it was Thursday you usually go
9. AP   no Thurs- Thurs- tomo-- tomorrow tomorrow
10. CP   that's Wednesday
11. AP   yeah that's right yeah
          (1.0)
12. CP   {dog enters room} that's him that's the one

AP introduces a new topic in T1 although, as for extract (*xix*) above, the precise focus of the topic is unclear, as indicated by the following turns. These consist of collaborative repair sequences, first around the issue of where he is going and then around the issue of the day that he goes. Following resolution of these, the topic is not developed further. There is a 1-second lapse in the conversation and AP starts a new topic relating to the dog that has entered the room. No strategies to maintain the topic are employed by CP. It would appear that limited maintenance of topic arises from difficulty in resolving multiple repair issues which are disruptive to development of the topic.

Topic maintenance can also be problematic if the person with aphasia opts to participate in conversation through the use of minimal turns. While this avoids exposing aphasic repair difficulties, as illustrated in extracts (*vii*) and (*xviii*) above, it also imposes the burden of maintaining the conversation upon the conversational partner.

Conversation analysis and its implications for therapy

In aphasia therapy, speech and language therapists frequently draw on a range of approaches to meet a particular person's needs. Two key approaches frequently drawn upon in a combination appropriate to a particular individual are:

1. impairment-focused therapy in which remediation of, or compensation for, the underlying language processing deficit is addressed;
2. communication-focused (or pragmatic) therapy in which compensation through the development of a range of communicative strategies in either the person with aphasia and/or his or her carers is addressed.

The implications of CA for each of these approaches will be considered in turn.

Impairment-focused therapy

In Part One, we discussed the strengths of a CN approach in motivating impairment-focused therapy. Using theoretical models of language processing, it is possible through CN assessment, to form a hypothesis about the processing impairments which underlie the individual person with aphasia's symptoms which can then be focused upon in therapy. As we discussed, however, the major weakness of a CN approach is that the tasks used in assessment and treatment are often heavily abstracted from the demands that the person with aphasia faces in his or her communicative environment.

From an assessment perspective, it is important to consider the impact that identified processing impairments have on the person with aphasia's ability to communicate in his or her social context. A CA allows an exploration of the impact of such processing impairments on interaction and so assists in identifying targets for therapy which will have the most functional impact for the individual.

From a therapy perspective, it is important to consider whether the outcome from impairment-focused therapy will result in an improvement beyond an increase in scores on CN assessments to improved interactional ability. Again, CA has a contribution to make here. For example, in the therapy study described by Best et al. (1997), discussed in Part One, JOW was taught the cognitive relay strategy of accessing the orthographic form to assist phonological retrieval. It is important, however, to consider whether he is able to use this strategy quickly enough in on-line conversation to resolve potential word finding difficulties or whether the conversational partner interjects to initiate collaborative repair beforehand. A conversation analysis would allow exploration of the effectiveness of the strategy in an interactional context. It may also indicate the need for some supplementary compensation-focused work in developing interactional strategies with the person with aphasia and his or her key conversational partners to accommodate use of the strategy in their interaction. The implications of CA for communication-focused therapy will be considered in the next section.

Communication-focused therapy

Communication-focused therapy (sometimes referred to as functional or pragmatic therapy) involves a shift from therapy aimed at improving the person with aphasia's production and comprehension of normal and 'correct' language structures. Instead remediation is concerned with the broader issue of optimal communication, with the use of all verbal and non-verbal resources available to maximise communication ability. While therapists have been using this type of approach in aphasia rehabilitation for a long time, the insights that CA can provide into aphasic interaction can strengthen such an approach.

A criticism which can be levelled at a pragmatic approach to therapy is that it focuses almost exclusively on the information transmission aspect of interaction, with little attention or value being placed on interaction which has a purely social function in which information transmission has only a minimal part to play. As has been highlighted by the work of Kagan and Gailey (1993) discussed earlier, however, it is loss of language as a social tool which has devastating effects on the person with aphasia and his or her family and there is a need to acknowledge this. CA provides an assessment tool to explore precisely how interaction between people with aphasia and their conversational partners is affected.

Frequently, communication-focused approaches to therapy involve teaching or encouraging the use of methods of communication which differ from that utilised in 'normal' interaction, for example the use of gesture, drawing, communication books and circumlocution. It is a common and frustrating experience for aphasia therapists to help people achieve a high level of competence in 'getting the message across' in the clinical situation, only to discover that none of the skills developed has generalised into the person's everyday life. CA provides us with some clues as to why this lack of generalisation is frequently experienced.

As highlighted in our discussion of repair, the CA literature has shown that revealing oneself as having a non-ordinary identity in conversation is interactionally delicate. People with aphasia are faced with this dilemma each time they start to speak and their 'non-ordinariness' is further displayed in the use of unusual communicative methods. For people who are still adapting and coming to terms with a new identity as aphasic speakers, it is not, therefore, surprising that they resist the use of strategies which further mark them as non-ordinary interactants, despite the fact that such strategies may allow them to be more successful communicators in terms of information transmission.

Another issue which may help explain the frequent lack of generalisation of strategies from the therapy room is the impact of the use of such strategies on conversational management procedures. First, the turn-taking mechanism operating in therapy tasks such as PACE activities (Davis and Wilcox, 1985) is very tolerant of delays while the person produces a turn using a non-verbal strategy. As has been highlighted in the discussion of turn-taking organisation above, however, delay is much less tolerated in peer conversation. Second, use of gesture, communication books or other alternative strategies involves more than the unilateral action of the person with aphasia as is shown in the following extract:

(xxi)
1. CP   there was a man sitting on a chair waiting for a haircut yes?
2. AP   mhm (erm 1.0) and erm *{gestures with left hand over head for 4 seconds from front to back}*
3. CP   when?
4. AP   *{repeats gesture with left hand quickly from front to back of head}*.
5. CP   when he cut it?
6. AP   yeah (I've got) mm well
7. CP   yes
8. AP   piece [ɒv] there *{gesturing over middle of head}* and piece o<ver there *{heheheheheheh}* ooh>
9. CP   <*{heheheheheheh}* this man> that was sitting waiting for his haircut?
10. AP   no
11. CP   no the w-

12. AP   the boy {points to CP}
13. CP   the boy
14. AP   erm {turns head and points to back and gestures over the top to the front
          with gesture repeated several times while CP takes next turn}
15. CP   when he had it cut?
16. AP   {gesture over the parting}
17. CP   through the middle?
18. AP   yes {points to CP}
19. CP   yes
20. AP   yeah
21. CP   when the man's seen he's having his hair cut through the middle
          what did he do?
          (1.5)
22. AP   nothing

In this extract in which AP is telling CP about an extract from a 'Mr Bean' comedy programme in which Mr Bean is pretending to be a barber, she uses gestures to convey that he cut a strip through the middle of the boy's hair. While the gestures that AP produces in this sequence contribute much to conveying this piece of information, the joint understanding that AP and CP reach also requires the collaborative contribution of CP to establish when it happened (T3 to T5 and T15), what happened (T17) and to whom it had happened (T9 to T13).

CA research into aphasic interaction has clearly demonstrated that conversation is a collaborative endeavour and the separation of the influence of the two interlocutors is arbitrary. This has implications for the manner in which communication-focused therapy is conducted. The utility of working with the person with aphasia's key conversational partners in strategy development (sometimes referred to as environmental therapy) has long been recognised (e.g. Newhoff, Bugbee and Ferreira, 1981; Miller 1989; Lesser and Algar, 1995). The findings of CA suggest that this should be taken one step further with development of strategies in partnership between the people with aphasia and their key conversational partners. Such an approach clearly has limitations in that it may only impact on interaction with the key conversational partner rather than equipping the person with aphasia to deal with a range of conversational partners in a variety of contexts. This has been addressed by Garrett, Beukelman and Low-Morrow (1989) in the intervention with a man described as having 'Broca's aphasia' who used written conversational control phrases (such as 'I'm changing topics', 'guess the word') as part of a multi-modal communication system to guide his conversational partners. Lesser and Algar (1995) described how a strategy advice book, developed on the basis of a joint CN–CA assessment for one woman's key conversational partner, was also read and acted upon by other friends and family members.

These discussions of the limitations of communicative strategies are not meant to imply that they have no role in aphasia intervention. Rather, we wish to highlight that CA research provides insights which might influence when such strategies are introduced, as well as informing which strategies may be useful for a particular interlocutor and how these strategies may best be developed. The ability of CA to reveal how people with aphasia and their conversational partners manage the manifestations of aphasia in interaction provides an extremely valuable method of assessment which can be used to motivate therapy, in which the outcome and effect on interaction of current strategies can be reviewed and the potential for development of further strategies explored.

An assessment tool which has been developed to assist in developing therapy in partnership with both the person with aphasia and his or her key conversational partners is the Conversation Analysis Profile for People with Aphasia (CAPPA; Whitworth, Perkins and Lesser, 1997). This uses a structured interview conducted with the key conversational partner and, where appropriate, the person with aphasia to supplement information obtained from analysis of a 10-minute sample of conversation. The information obtained from both sources provides a starting point for the therapist to negotiate between the person with aphasia and his or her key conversational partner about potential modifications to their current interactional management. The information gleaned from the interview empowers the couple to set the therapy agenda, rather than strategies being 'prescribed' as good or bad by the therapist.

Undertaking a conversation analysis

Undertaking a conversation analysis involves three main steps. The first of these is to collect a recording of conversation on which to undertake the analysis. The second step involves transcription of a sample of data. The final stage is deciding the focus of the analysis and carrying out the analysis itself. A brief outline of these steps is provided below.

Recording

The purpose of obtaining a recording for CA is to obtain an interaction which is naturally occurring, in order to provide as much information about the functioning of the person in his or her social context. The first decision is who the conversational partner(s) should be. As has emerged from the CA and aphasia literature reviewed above, conversation is a collaborative achievement and very different interactional outcomes may be found for the same person with aphasia with different conversational partners. Most frequently, the person with aphasia's partner or main carer will be chosen, as this will be the person with whom he or she has most interaction. If, however, goals of intervention are more specific, recording with different conversational partners may be more useful. For example, if someone reports a particular interactional difficulty in a multi-party setting, such as a family gathering or with friends, a recording in this situation would be most informative to intervention. For an individual living in a residential home, a recording of interactions with staff may be useful.

A further decision is where to make the recording. As the goal is to record a conversation which would have happened anyway, recording in the home environment is preferable to recording in the clinic. The latter context is more likely to give rise to a contrived conversation 'performed' for the tape recorder or video. The practicality of recording in the home environment will depend on the individual therapist's work context.

Where it is possible to make a recording at home, it is important to stress that what you are trying to capture is a conversation that would have happened anyway. A common response is for couples to say that they never talk. Usually, through discussion, it is possible to establish a time when they are more likely to talk, for example, over the main meal of the day or when one of them has returned home after being out. If possible, it is helpful to leave the recording equipment for them to switch on at a time when they are likely to talk. The recording should be made without the therapist being present, as the presence of an observing third person will influence the interaction. They should also be reassured that they do not have to talk continuously.

The choice of video or audio recording will be influenced by a number of factors. The most obvious of these is the availability of equipment. The advantage of video recording is that non-verbal language is also captured for analysis and this will be particularly important for a recording of a person with severely limited verbal output. Video is, however, more obtrusive and some people may not feel comfortable being video-recorded. In these cases, more naturalistic data may be collected through an audio recording.

Ten minutes of interaction provide a large amount of data for analysis. It is preferable to collect more, if this is possible, since there may be lapses in the conversation. Where the person and his or her conversational partner feel uncomfortable about being recorded, it may be preferable to discard the first part of the recording. Finally, if the analysis is to be focused on a particular aspect of interaction, for example, collaborative repair sequences, it may be necessary to have a longer recording in order to capture enough examples of the focus of the analysis.

It is important to ensure confidentiality for any recordings that are made. Written permission for video recording should be obtained, with the purpose of the recording being specified. Furthermore, for both audio and video recording, all conversational partners should be given the opportunity to wipe the recording or part of the recording, without being required to give an explanation, before it has been viewed or heard.

Transcription

Transcription for the purposes of CA differs from that of transcription used for other analytic purposes (for example phonetic or syntactic analysis) in that it needs to capture features relevant to the interaction. The first major difference, therefore, is that all conversational partners' conversational turns need to be transcribed, rather than simply focusing on the production of the person with the language disorder. Second, the minutiae of interaction such as overlaps, filled and unfilled pauses and dysfluencies are included as they may have important interactional consequences. For video data, transcription of non-verbal features may also be important. A set of transcription conventions originally developed by Jefferson is widely used in CA and a modified set of these conventions which we have used in the extracts in this book is provided in Appendix C. As noted by Lesser and Milroy (1993: p. 172) there is no such thing as an absolutely complete or correct transcription. The level of detail required will be influenced by the focus of the analysis.

Transcription is time-consuming. It is necessary to decide whether to transcribe a continuous stretch of conversation or whether to transcribe more selectively. For a continuous transcription, 5–10 minutes will provide a wealth of information. This type of approach is useful to secure an overall picture of the interaction and how aphasia is being handled by the conversational partners. If, however, you wish to focus upon a particular aspect of the interaction, for example, collaborative repair sequences as we mentioned above, selective transcription may be more appropriate in which the recording is scanned for the particular interactional occurrences of interest.

Analysis

Since conversation analysis is a data-driven, qualitative process, there is no prescribed way in which to undertake the analysis. The first step is to look at the transcript and listen to or watch the recording to try and identify patterns in the interaction which are of particular interest. It may then be fruitful to focus on conversational management features which are of particular relevance to that particular individual. The discussion above of turn-taking, repair and topic management should assist in this process. It may also be helpful to focus on the manifestations of specific linguistic impairments and their impact on interaction. Lesser and Milroy (1993: pp. 324ff) provide a checklist of conversational abilities and the CAPPA (Whitworth, Perkins and Lesser, 1997) provides a structured form to guide the search for evidence of interactional features and their subsequent conversational management.

CA has almost exclusively focused on qualitative analysis with a rejection of quantification. Schegloff (1988: p. 136) states that 'social action done through talk is organised and orderly on a case by case basis, and not only as a matter of rule or statistical regularity'. The major danger of quantifying conversational behaviour is that CA's central notion of evidence from the sequential context is lost as items are removed from their context for counting. The collaborative nature of interaction is particularly vulnerable to being lost if, in the quantification, the actions of the two interlocutors are separated out from each other. More recently some researchers have acknowledged, however, that for some purposes quantitative analysis may have a useful supplementary role to qualitative analysis (Schegloff, 1993). For its validity the analyst must be cognisant of the limitations of quantification and design the analysis to be sensitive to the sequential context by building it on the back of qualitative single-instance analysis. Aphasia assessment is one context in which quantification would appear to play a useful supplementary role to qualitative analysis. As outlined by Lesser and Milroy (1993), although qualitative analysis offers a basis for intervention in accurately identifying areas to target in therapy, quantification has the major advantage of facilitating comparison, which is important in the evaluation of the effectiveness of therapy.

Preliminary work (Crockford and Lesser, 1994; Perkins, 1995a, b) has shown that quantification of some conversational behaviours can be useful in comparing aphasic conversations provided it is interpreted within the findings of qualitative analyses. If CA is to be used for test–retest purposes, it is necessary to address the criticism made by Manochiopinig, Sheard and Reed (1992) that assessments which are based on the observation of a conversation are subject to sampling error and are, therefore, unsuitable for the precise measurement of performance over time.

A recently completed research project (Perkins, Lesser and Milroy, 1998) addressed this issue using a range of quantitative and qualitative analyses to examine the variation in conversational management between conversations of eight people with stable aphasia and their relatives on four consecutive weeks. Significant within-participant variation was found for the quantitative analyses undertaken, indicating that use of the quantitative measures could not, on their own, be taken as an indication of change over time since this could simply reflect conversation-to-conversation variation. Where a statistically significant change is still detected, this provides evidence for a real effect of therapy. In a second phase of the study which investigated change in the conversations of people with aphasia in the phase of spontaneous recovery, quantification of the proportion of major turns involved in collaborative repair was found to be sensitive to recovery between three months and seven months post-stroke even after adjustment for conversation-to-conversation variation.

The qualitative analyses undertaken for the study supported the use of CA as a tool to detect change over time. In the first phase of the project which examined people with stable aphasia, reliability was found in both the interactional challenges experienced as a consequence of aphasia and the interactional mechanisms employed to deal with these over the four repeated data collections (Perkins, Crisp and Walshaw, 1999). This is an important finding which supports the validity of qualitative CA as an assessment method for planning intervention. In the second phase of the project investigating change with spontaneous recovery, the qualitative analyses were able to demonstrate change over time. Analyses of both self repair and collaborative repair were particularly sensitive to change in both the nature of trouble sources and mode of resolution. Change in topic management and turn taking was also detectable for two participants. Booth and Perkins (1999) describe a single case study which illustrates the use of qualitative conversation analysis to both motivate intervention and demonstrate the effect of therapy.

Having provided a brief introduction to CA and its implications for aphasia management, we now provide three further cases for you to work through. These follow the same pattern as the first three cases in the book but, in addition to being asked to plan and interpret psycholinguistic assessment, you are also asked to plan and interpret CA assessment before considering how you might develop intervention.

Case 4
Mrs EM

When you work through this case remember to read the information first and then write down your own interpretation and ideas before you turn the page to read ours.

Initial impressions

Read through the case description and think about what the important features are that will guide your selection of assessments.

Case description

EM is a housewife who lives at home with her retired husband. They have four adult sons, one of whom lives locally. EM had 9 years of education and worked in the local glass factory before having her children. She is left-handed.

When EM was 65 she suffered a left cerebrovascular accident (CVA) and was admitted to hospital with a right hemiplegia and aphasia. She received physiotherapy and speech and language therapy and this continued on a weekly basis after discharge from hospital. Six and a half months after the CVA she fell and broke her hip. As a consequence she was immobile and unable to attend for speech and language therapy at the local hospital. She was therefore referred to the community therapist.

The referral reported that EM's major difficulty was word-finding. This caused her a high level of frustration in conversation, to an extent that she would give up trying to communicate what she had been attempting. On picture naming EM's most common error was that she could not retrieve the word. She also produced a small number of phonemic and semantic errors. In her functional communication there was no evidence of comprehension difficulties. She reported that she no longer wrote letters.

Your initial hypotheses

Using the information given in the case description, consider the possible loci of EM's impairments. Given the limited information that you have, you may have several tentative hypotheses (the number of spaces provided is not intended as a guide). What is the justification for each of the hypotheses? What further information would you require to confirm or reject each of these?

If you want to keep the book unmarked, use the photocopiable sheets on pp. 232–239.

EM's difficulties compromise the

_____

Justification for this is that

_____
_____
_____
_____
_____
_____
_____

EM's difficulties compromise the

_____

Justification for this is that

_____
_____
_____
_____
_____
_____
_____

EM's difficulties compromise the

_____

Justification for this is that

_____
_____
_____
_____
_____
_____

EM's difficulties compromise the

_____

Justification for this is that

_____
_____
_____
_____
_____
_____
_____

EM's difficulties compromise the

_____

Justification for this is that

_____
_____
_____
_____
_____
_____
_____

What other factors need to be taken into consideration in planning assessments for EM?

_____

_____

_____

_____

_____

_____

_____

_____

_____

Our hypotheses

> When you have completed your hypotheses, compare them to our suggestions. As you can see, it is not possible to propose firm hypotheses, but tentative possibilities can guide the selection of assessments, and each assessment should contribute to the identification of the level of deficit.

EM's difficulties compromise the semantic system.

Justification for this is that she produces semantic errors in naming and shows a failure in lexical retrieval. This is only one possible locus of impairment (see below). Further assessment of semantic processing through comprehension tasks and perhaps written output should help to decide between the possibilities.

EM's difficulties compromise the phonological output lexicon or access to it.

Justification for this is that she demonstrates failures in lexical retrieval. This impairment could also account for the small number of semantic and phonemic paraphasias produced. It is necessary to assess further to distinguish between an impairment at this level and one involving the semantic system.

EM's difficulties compromise the phonological assembly buffer.

Justification for this is that she produces a small number of phonemic paraphasias. This is not the only hypothesis for this deficit. Impairment to the phonological output lexicon could also account for this error type.

The assessments used will need to take into consideration EM's high level of frustration. It will be important for her not to experience a high level of failure in the tasks. Assessments will therefore need to be carefully balanced so that she experiences success at tasks.

There is very little information provided about EM's production in the written modality except for her statement that she is no longer able to write letters. Comparison of written and spoken output could be useful in determining the locus of impairment as well as investigating possible intact abilities to harness in therapy.

Your selection of assessments

Now that you have some initial hypotheses about the loci of impairments, plan the types of assessment tasks that you would employ to test out your hypotheses. We have provided spaces for several assessments, but this does not mean that we expect you to use the exact number. You will find that selection of one assessment will be influenced by the potential findings of previous ones carried out.

Assessment

Justification for selection

Assessment

Justification for selection

Assessment

Justification for selection

Assessment

Justification for selection

Assessment

Justification for selection

Assessment

Justification for selection

Our selection of assessments

> Now you have selected possible assessments compare them to the suggestions that we have made. Remember that there is no single right way of assessing someone using a psycholinguistic perspective. You should, however, be able to justify the need for each of the assessments in testing out specific hypotheses regarding the locus of impairment. If you selected different assessments, look at the assessments that were selected and work out the rationale behind this choice.

Assessment: Word–picture matching assessments in both spoken and written modality. Possible assessments that could be used are PALPA 47 *Spoken word–picture matching* and PALPA 48 *Written word–picture matching*. Alternatives include ADACB S2 *Auditory word–picture matching* and ADACB S2Wr *Written word–picture matching*. Another semantic assessment for which comparison of picture, spoken and written input can be made is the Pyramids and Palm Trees Test.

Justification for selection: These assessments would allow the investigation of whether EM has a semantic impairment which is compromising spoken output and giving rise to her word-finding difficulties. Examination in both modalities would allow the identification of a central semantic impairment, in which case she would be expected to perform equivalently in both modalities. If she was only impaired in one modality, this would indicate that she has an impairment in accessing the semantic system from one modality. In this case, a semantic locus of impairment could not account for her impairment in lexical retrieval.

Assessment: Assessment of semantic processing for low imageability items. Possible assessments include PALPA 49 *Auditory synonym judgement* and PALPA 50 *Written synonym judgement* or ADACB S1 *Auditory synonym matching* and ADACB S1Wr *Written synonym judgement*.

Justification for selection: If EM performs at a high level on word–picture matching assessments of semantic processing, investigation of her semantic knowledge for low imageability items may be useful to check whether she has an impairment of abstract semantics. Comparison of performance in auditory and written modalities would allow identification of a central semantic impairment, in which case she would be expected to perform equivalently in both modalities. As we noted in respect of the word–picture matching tests, if she was only impaired in one modality, this would indicate that she has an impairment in accessing the semantic system, in this case for low imageability words.

Assessment: Assessment of oral and written picture naming controlled for word frequency, such as PALPA 54 *Picture naming × frequency* or its precursor the *Kay Naming Test*.

Justification for selection: An effect of word frequency has been associated with an impairment in access to the phonological output lexicon (Kay and Ellis, 1989; Ellis, Franklin and Crerar, 1994). Comparison of oral and written naming will identify any effect of mode of output on EM's performance. If EM shows equivalent performance in both assessments, this would support the hypothesis of a central semantic impairment, or a problem which implicates access to both the phonological output lexicon and the graphemic output lexicon. If she shows written naming that is superior to spoken naming, this would indicate that her word-finding difficulty involves the phonological output lexicon, and that her main input to the graphemic output lexicon is direct from semantics rather than mediated through the phonological output lexicon.

Assessment: Repetition assessment. Numerous assessments could be selectively used to investigate the effect of word length (e.g. PALPA 7 *Repetition: syllable length*), frequency and imageability (e.g. PALPA 9 *Repetition: imageability × frequency*) or lexicality (e.g. PALPA 8 *Repetition: non-words*). ADACB L2 *Repetition of words* combines examination of word length, frequency and imageability.

Justification for selection: A repetition assessment will provide useful information to tease out the specific locus or loci of the phonological errors reported in her picture-naming performance. If these are arising because of an impairment involving the phonological output lexicon, then repetition may be intact, as she may be able to utilise the non-lexical route converting phonological input to output. If she makes phonological errors in repetition and shows a length effect with more errors on longer words, this may indicate involvement of the phonological assembly buffer.

Assessment results

> Now read through the results of the assessments that we actually carried out.

PALPA 47 Spoken word–picture matching and PALPA 48 Written word–picture matching

EM made no errors on these assessments.

PALPA 49 Auditory synonym judgement and PALPA 50 Written synonym judgement

EM scored 56 out of 60 on the spoken version and 54 out of 60 on the written version. This falls below the performance of normal control subjects. All except one of the errors involved low imageability items. All the errors were false-positives (accepting non-synonym pairs as synonyms).

Kay Naming Test (revised): Oral naming and written naming

When asked to name orally, EM made 53 out of 75 correct responses within 5 seconds. She named a further 11 items after this time period. She made two semantic errors and had nine failures to name. Within her attempts she produced circumlocutions, semantic associates and six phonemic paraphasias, all of which were self-corrected. There was an effect of word frequency with 88% of high frequency items correct in comparison to 48% of low frequency items.

When asked to write the names of the pictures, EM demonstrated superior written retrieval in comparison to spoken retrieval, with 70 out of 75 immediately correct responses. For three of the low-frequency items, there was a delay of over 5 seconds before she correctly wrote the names, and for a further two items there was a failure to name.

PALPA 9 Repetition: imageability × frequency

EM repeated all of the items without error. Her performance therefore fell within the normal range.

Your interpretation of the results of the assessments

What do the assessment results mean? Map out your hypotheses of the locus or loci of EM's production deficit based on these findings, using the diagram of the model. Indicate also what processes seem to be preserved and which levels you are uncertain about from the assessment results so far. Note down the justification in support of your hypotheses.

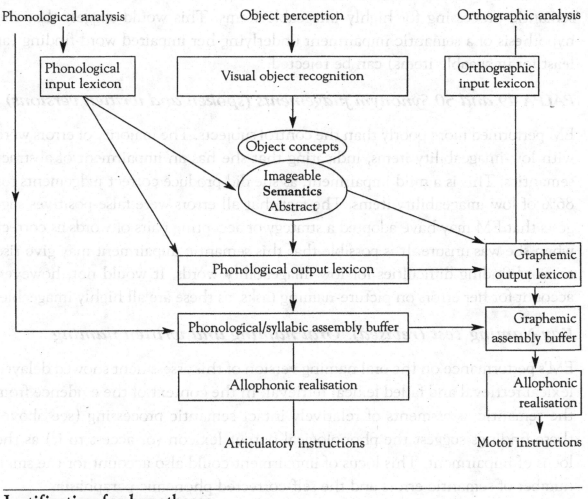

Justification for hypotheses

Our interpretation of the results of the assessments

> Now read through our interpretation of the psycholinguistic findings.

PALPA 47 and 48 Word–picture matching (spoken and written versions)

EM made no errors on these tasks, indicating that she has relatively intact semantic processing for highly imageable items. This would suggest that the hypothesis of a semantic impairment underlying her impaired word-finding (at least for imageable items) can be rejected.

PALPA 49 and 50 Synonym judgements (spoken and written versions)

EM performed more poorly than the control subjects. The majority of errors were with low-imageability items, indicating that she has an impairment of abstract semantics. This is a mild impairment, as she did produce correct judgements for 86% of low imageability items. The fact that all errors were false-positives suggests that EM may have adopted a strategy of accepting pairs of words as correct when she was unsure. It is possible that this semantic impairment may give rise to word-finding difficulties for low-imageability words. It would not, however, account for her errors on picture-naming tasks, as these are all highly imageable.

Kay Naming Test (revised): Oral naming and written naming

EM's performance on the oral naming version of this assessment showed delayed lexical retrieval and failed lexical retrieval. In the context of the evidence from the semantic assessments of relatively intact semantic processing (see above) these findings suggest the phonological output lexicon (or access to it) as the locus of impairment. This locus of impairment could also account for the small number of semantic errors and the self-corrected phonemic paraphasias.

These hypotheses are supported by EM's better performance on the written version of this assessment. The ability to retrieve lexical items through the graphic modality, which she could not name orally, supports the hypothesis that EM has access to the semantic representations. Although retrieval from the graphemic output lexicon on the test was not perfect, the superior performance of written over oral naming indicates a greater impairment in retrieval from the phonological output lexicon.

PALPA 9 Repetition: imageability × frequency

EM's performance on this assessment indicates that she has only a mild impairment in phonological processing which does not compromise her ability to repeat words in isolation. This is supported by her ability to self-correct the phonological errors she makes in picture naming and in spontaneous speech. It is therefore unlikely that she is impaired in respect of the phonological assembly buffer.

Conversation analysis: selecting parameters for assessment

We will ask you shortly what inferences for therapy you might draw from the psycholinguistic findings. Meanwhile from the results of the cognitive neuropsychological assessment and the information given in the case description, consider what analyses of conversation you would like to undertake to gain information to guide therapy.

Conversational data to be collected

Analysis

Justification for selection

Analysis

Justification for selection

Analysis

Justification for selection

Our selection of parameters for conversation analysis

> Now that you have selected some possible analyses, compare them to the suggestions that we have made. If you selected different analyses, look at the ones that we selected and work out the rationale behind this choice.

Conversational data to be collected: To make decisions about the most useful context (situations and conversational partners) in which to record conversation, it is necessary to collect information about EM's most frequent conversational partners and communicative situations. The case description informs us that she is housebound and this therefore limits the context to the home. As she lives with her husband, he is likely to be the most frequent conversational partner and therefore analysis of EM's conversation with him would be useful. It may also be useful to obtain a recording of a multi-party conversation, perhaps when family and friends visit, to investigate whether this context is more difficult for her

Analysis: Turn-taking.

Justification for selection: Psycholinguistic assessment shows that EM has a lexical retrieval deficit with delayed and failed lexical retrieval on a picture-naming assessment. This impairment may influence EM's ability to take her turns in conversation without a delay and to complete her turns. She may lose the floor to her conversational partners if she has long silences in her turns as she tries to retrieve words. An analysis of turn-taking would therefore be useful to see whether and how this impairment handicaps EM in conversation.

Analysis: Distribution of conversational turns between conversational partner.

Justification for selection: In the case description, we were told that EM suffered a high level of frustration from her word-finding difficulties, which resulted in her giving up attempts to communicate. It would therefore be useful to get a measure of the number of minimal and major turns produced by EM and her conversational partners to establish how the conversational burden is shared.

Analysis: Repair patterns.

Justification for selection: EM's linguistic impairments will give rise to breakdowns in the conversation. An analysis of both self-repair and collaborative repair patterns will allow an examination of current strategies used by both EM and her conversational partners to resolve these difficulties. Such information is potentially useful for the development of more effective communication strategies for both the aphasic person and her conversational partners.

Results of the conversation analyses

> Now read through the findings of the analyses undertaken.

Conversational data collected: Although EM's most frequent conversational partner was her husband, the couple reported that it was not a normal activity to sit and talk together and they were reluctant to make a recording. EM reported that her male cousin who visited her several times a week to have a chat was her most frequent conversational partner. EM was therefore left with a tape recorder and she switched it on for one of these visits. No recording of a multi-party conversation was made, as EM reported that the majority of visits that she had were with one person. A recording of EM talking to a speech and language therapist on her first visit was also available for analysis. This was analysed as it was felt that it was potentially useful to compare EM's conversational abilities with different conversational partners. Twelve minutes of each conversation (excluding lapses in the interaction) were selected, thus providing samples of the same size to facilitate comparison between the two conversations.

Analysis of turn-taking: An examination of turn-taking in both the conversation with her cousin and the conversation with the speech and language therapist demonstrated her ability to take a turn without gap or overlap. EM's word-finding difficulties did, however, result in long filled and unfilled pauses within her turns. In 14 (26%) of her major turns in the conversation with her relative and three (4%) of her major turns in the conversation with the speech and language therapist, the conversational partner initiated a turn before EM had completed her turn. An example of this from the conversation with the therapist is given below:

1. EM and er:: (2:0)
2. CP so you've got another room down here as well as your kitchen and your lounge?
3. EM yeah er and er (2:0)
4. CP right
5. EM mm

It therefore appears that pauses which arise during lexical search (see T1 and T3) make EM vulnerable to the loss of the conversational floor as her conversational partners do not tolerate long pauses.

Analysis of the distribution of conversational turns between conversational partners: In the conversation with her cousin, EM was observed to exploit the use of minimal turns to pass the conversational floor back to her cousin without producing major turns. This is illustrated in the following extract:

1. CP   so I just took it in he says that's all <put> your name on there I says that's it he says that's in it he says that's it
2. EM   <mm>
3. EM   aha
4. CP   I says why and then I got something for the the dole for the council <offices> I take that up and all I says there you are fill that in I says and I'll tell you all you want to know
5. EM   <mm mm>
6. EM   {hehe}
         (1.0)
7. CP   why you can't understand it when you're <2 syll.>
8. EM   <well its its> its [tə]
9. CP   I must be <thick> never mind Jean=
10. EM   <mhm>
11. EM   ={hehehehe<hehehehehe} eee:>
12. CP   <aye you cannot understand> half of them
13. EM   aye
         (2.3)
14. CP   but er y'know we used to get a a rebate from Scotland
15. EM   mhm
16. CP   y'know off the rent
17. EM   mhm
18. CP   well that's been stopped 'cause we cannot get a get a rise on our pensions
19. EM   mhm
20. CP   so I'm not allowed that anymore <so> that's stopped it's finished
21. EM   <tsk>
22. EM   {hehehe}

EM repeatedly produced acknowledgement tokens and laughter, which allowed her to participate without requiring the production of more linguistically challenging major turns. T6 and T13 are of particular note as, following EM's minimal turn, there was a lapse in the conversation. She did not, however, take these opportunities to take the conversational floor. Instead the cousin reinitiated after each lapse. The outcome of this was that he took a more dominant role in the conversation with little input from EM. In T8 EM does attempt to produce a major turn, but her cousin produced a further major turn before it was completed, resulting in a failure in EM's attempt to contribute to the conversation. This pattern was reflected in quantification of the proportion of major turns produced by each of the participants, with 30% being produced by EM and 70% being produced by her cousin.

Analysis of EM's conversation with the speech and language therapist did not reveal the same pattern of reliance on minimal turns to participate in conversation. As illustrated in the following extract, in this conversation EM successfully took the conversational floor and contributed major turns (see T2, T6 and T11):

1.   CP   your husband seems a really good help though
2.   EM   well that's that's just God er erm got here is oh God is (1 syll.) that's [bɛtənt] me down
3.   CP   that's getting you <down>
4.   EM   <yes> yeah
5.   CP   what er what
6.   EM   well I mean it's er (1.3) {hehe} it's oh it's (0.7)
7.   CP   yeah it's just sort of being (0.6) you're sort of stuck <here> and you can't get out
8.   EM   <yeah>
9.   EM   yeah
10.   CP   yeah
11.   EM   yeah and there's this sort of (1.5) everything in its er look at this

This extract illustrates that, while EM did run into linguistic difficulty when she contributed major turns to the conversation, she was nevertheless able to contribute actively to the development of the topic. In contrast to the more passive role that she took in the conversation with her cousin, quantitative analysis revealed that the conversational floor was shared more equally in the conversation with the speech and language therapist: EM produced 53% of the major turns and the therapist produced 47%.

Analysis of repair patterns: In both of the conversations analysed there were sequences of repair work carried out collaboratively between EM and her conversational partners. These could be seen to deal with trouble sources in the conversation which arose from EM's lexical retrieval deficit. While in the conversation with her cousin there were three collaborative repair sequences, in the conversation with the therapist there were 18 sequences. Although less repair work could be expected in EM's conversation with her relative, given the fact that she produced a smaller proportion of major turns in this conversation (see analysis of distribution of major turns), this does not account for the magnitude of the difference. A further factor that appears to influence the quantity of collaborative repair in the two conversations is the differential treatment of potentially problematic turns by the two conversational partners. It was reported in the analysis of turn-taking that EM lost her turn before completion in 26% of cases in the conversation with her cousin, in contrast to only 4% of cases in the conversation with the speech and language therapist. There is evidence in the conversations of different interactional patterns being employed to cope with EM's linguistic impairments. In the conversation with her cousin, EM's potentially problematic turns were glossed over before completion, with her cousin taking the conversational floor and continuing to develop the topic. This is shown in the following extract:

1. CP ...and I thought the way she was talking I thought she might have been away about a fortnight
2. EM no she was [wə] she was supposed to er (0.6) I've forgotten but she was but she was (1.6)
3. CP I was talking to her at the butcher's down the bottom

This contrasts with the greater use of collaborative repair between EM and the speech and language therapist to resolve EM's problematic turns, as is illustrated in the two extracts discussed below in relation to collaborative repair patterns.

An examination of the trouble sources that gave rise to collaborative repair work showed that some repairs dealt with failure in retrieval of specific lexical items. Three involved the clarification of a deictic referring expression that EM had used as a strategy to compensate for lexical retrieval deficits. Another repair sequence dealt with clarification of a pointing response that EM had used to compensate for a word-finding failure. A further sequence dealt with clarification where EM had used writing in the air for the word that she was unable to access through the spoken modality. An example is given below from the conversation with the therapist:

1.   EM   and er there's [tstss] (2:1) [s::] {ha} (4:0) {EM *fingerspells the word bungalow*}
2.   CP   oh it's a low it's <a> bungalow
3.   EM   <yeah>
4.   EM   [brʊn] bungalow
5.   CP   oh that'll be a lot better for you

All of these demonstrate the collaborative nature of the repair work with the unimpaired conversational partner building on the strategies that EM had developed (gesture, writing, etc.) to achieve an understanding of the problematic turn. In addition, there were eight repair sequences in which the work could be seen to be concerned with establishment of a general understanding of EM's turn. These arose because EM produced turns with several clauses abandoned because of failures in lexical retrieval. These turns were often lexically empty and repair was initiated by the conversational partner either asking specific questions to help achieve an understanding or by picking up the gist and formulating an interpretation of the problematic turn. Although on some occasions this resulted in fast resolution, some repair work resulted in more protracted resolution over several turns. An example of this from the conversation with the therapist is given below:

1.   CP   so what did they say?
2.   EM   so I have to wait 'til we (1:5) to when I know (1:4) er (1:2) you see have took me and I could have rode and I said n-n- no not (1:0) <(1 syll.)>
3.   CP   <oh> in the wheelchair to the General?
              (1:7)
4.   CP   what your husband was going to push you there?
5.   EM   no she's going to no because she were going to put er (1:3) hhh no because it was [kət kət] (2:0) mhm (2:8) they could have put this in the [dʒə] in the [drə]

6. CP   in the ambulance?
7. EM   mhm
8. CP   yeah but there is no way that you could have got that there without an ambulance is there?
9. EM   yeah that's right

Planning initial intervention

> From the findings of these assessment results it is proposed that EM has a mild abstract semantic impairment and an impairment involving the phonological output lexicon. The conversation analysis demonstrates that the latter impairment significantly impacts on conversational ability. The effect that this has on EM's conversation is influenced in turn by the strategies of both EM and her conversational partners. What therapy would you derive from the findings of the psycholinguistic assessments and the conversation analysis?

Our suggestions for initial intervention

Now that you have thought about some possible interventions, compare them with our suggestions. Remember that these are only tentative ideas and may differ from yours. Both your and our ideas may be appropriate. The important issue is that intervention should be motivated by theoretical principles.

EM has difficulty in accessing representations in the phonological output lexicon. This impacts significantly on her participation in conversation, to a greater degree than might be predicted from her performance on a formal picture naming test. To some extent this may be associated with the mild disorder of abstract semantics which was identified, although no direct evidence of this was found in the conversations. The access difficulty is a source of major frustration to her. A twofold approach in intervention may therefore be indicated: direct therapy for the deficit and indirect therapy involving both her and her conversational partners in achieving more effective communication.

Since it has been proposed that high-frequency words are easier to access because they have higher resting levels of activation than words of low frequency, one approach to therapy could be to raise the threshold of representations in the lexicon by massive practice. Output could be achieved by any input including repetition and reading. Since thresholds of individual lexical items will be being raised, an item-specific effect of therapy would be predicted. It will therefore be necessary to select treatment items which have the greatest relevance to EM. Hillis and Caramazza (1994) describe a therapy programme for a patient with impairment involving the phonological output lexicon, which worked on this principle using a hierarchy of sentence completion tasks with an initial phoneme cue and spoken word as a model. An item-specific effect was found.

An alternative impairment-focused approach would be to use a cognitive relay strategy in which EM is encouraged to use orthographic/graphemic information to increase the activation at the phonological output lexicon. Her superior performance on written, in comparison to oral, naming, indicates that this would be an appropriate avenue to explore; this is supported by her spontaneous use of a spelling-out strategy identified from the conversation analysis. It may therefore be possible to teach her to access first-letter information to increase activation to the lexical phonological form and cue herself. Bruce and Howard (1987) describe therapy which achieved this outcome for one of the patients treated. Alternatively, it may be possible to teach her to visualise the orthographic form of the word and read it back. Further assessment of reading and writing ability would be advisable before pursuing this approach. If it proved feasible, however, it has the advantage of being generalisable to retrieval of all words.

The conversation analysis is particularly revealing of the effect of EM's retrieval problems and the probable cause of her frustrations. Her delays, repetitions and abandoned clauses contribute to different patterns in the two conversations. Her cousin is intolerant of delays and continues without engaging in collaborative repairs to any significant extent; this results in the majority of EM's turns being minor ones with loss of the conversational floor. In contrast, the therapist tolerates delays and there are frequent collaborative sequences, with, as a consequence, a more balanced sharing of major turns. Following EM's multiple attempts at self-repair with little lexical content and short abandoned clauses, the conversational partners engage in collaborative sequences aimed at achieving a general understanding of the topic in which EM is engaged. The cousin could be encouraged to adopt this strategy, and ask questions and formulate interpretations, rather than glossing over EM's problems. The comparison of the two conversations suggests that EM's reliance on minimal turns is a consequence of the joint activity between her and her cousin rather than an avoidance strategy, as she takes a full share of major turns in the conversation with the therapist.

These findings have two major implications. First, work on turn-taking to encourage EM's conversational partners to allow her more time to produce her conversational turn could be expected to enable her to take a more active role in conversation. In view of her frequent delays, she could be encouraged to use floor-holding techniques, such as eye gaze, gesture and filling of pauses (Ahlsen, 1985). Second, work could be undertaken to equip EM and her conversational partner with more effective strategies to be able to undertake collaborative repair. Specific communicative strategies could be encouraged in EM. It was noted that she used writing in the air as a means of helping her word retrieval. This could be developed to be used more frequently, with her conversational partner being taught to allow time for EM to use the strategy. A framework for circumlocutions could be developed which would enable her to supply information more systematically and lead either to her retrieval of the target word or to the interlocutor's recognition of the meaning. Reinforcement of strategies taught could be achieved through the use of information booklets (Lesser and Algar, 1995).

Developing the hypotheses

Remember that the results of assessment (and of intervention) feed back into developing the hypotheses you initially made. There may also be gaps in your interpretation, which the results have revealed. Use this page to write down what further investigations you might wish to consider to develop your hypotheses, some of which may depend on EM's response to therapy. **Cover up the next page (which has our suggestions) until you have written yours down.**

Our suggestions for developing the hypotheses

> Now read through the suggestions that we have made and compare them with your own.

If, as noted earlier, a strategy is to be considered of teaching EM to visualise the orthographic form of the word and 'read' it back, it will be necessary to establish the integrity of her orthographic input lexicon. PALPA 25 *Visual lexical decision: imageability × frequency* and PALPA 27 *Visual lexical decision: spelling-sound regularity* may illuminate this.

EM's lexical retrieval deficit impacts significantly on her conversational ability to a greater degree than might be predicted from her performance on a formal picture naming test. Whitworth (1994, 1995) has demonstrated that anomia at a sentence level may also arise as a consequence of an impairment to thematic role processing. It may therefore be useful to investigate whether EM has an impairment to this process. Thematic Roles in Production (TRIP; Whitworth, 1996) would permit investigation of thematic role processing in production. Examination of the effect of reversibility on comprehension using PALPA 55 *Auditory sentence comprehension* would also provide information about thematic role processing. A comparison of results from both could permit inferences about the supra-modal nature of any difficulties across production and comprehension.

Case 5
Mrs JN

When you work through this case remember to read the information first and then write down your own interpretation and ideas before you turn the page to read ours.

Initial impressions

> Read through the case description and think about what the important features are that will guide your selection of assessments.

Case description

JN is a retired factory seamstress. She is a widow who lives on her own, but has a daughter and a sister nearby. She is a sociable person, although her relatives have noticed that she is having some trouble with remembering things. She has a history of mild epilepsy, now no longer requiring drug control.

At the age of 80, she was found collapsed and unconscious at home (coma scale 8/14). On arrival at the hospital she was making incomprehensible sounds. No lesion showed on a CT scan, but she was diagnosed as having suffered a stroke with dysphasia.

Four days later she was sitting up, and responding appropriately in short sentences with some jargon speech. Her response when asked to write her signature was to write 'Week if I veek', but the following day she wrote her signature correctly on request, although expressing some uncertainty as to whether it was correct. She was unable to name drawings of objects, apparently not recognising some, but giving semantic associates of others. On PALPA 47 *Spoken word–picture matching* she scored 14 out of 40 with 13 close semantic errors, six distant semantic errors and seven visual errors. She appeared to be unable to read words for meaning, i.e. in matching written words with objects.

Two weeks later, able to walk and without any hemiparesis, she was discharged home, with her daughter and sister in close attendance. This was the

150

daughter and sister's first experience of stroke, and they were keen to know more about aphasia and to help her. They commented that she was sometimes forgetful and a little confused, and that they sometimes had to repeat themselves before she seemed to understand what they were saying.

By 3 months post-onset, her speech was fluent without jargon, although she still had difficulty finding some words. She was coping well at home, although still showing mild confusions. As an example of this, her sister described how she had given her grandson a £10 note instead of £1, as she had forgotten that £1 notes have been replaced with coins, and was distressed on discovering her mistake; on another occasion she offered tea to a visitor, and then made coffee for her. She also showed some perseveration of thought in the clinic, for example, when asked to write 'tree' she wrote 'pencil' (she was writing with one) and then attempted to correct this, resulting in 'pin'.

Five months post-onset, she had a minor fall and was readmitted to hospital for a checkup. A CT scan at this stage showed three infarcts: a left fronto-temporal, thought to be associated with the cause of her first admission, and more recent left and right parieto-occipital infarcts.

Your initial hypotheses

Using the information given in the case description, consider the possible loci of JN's impairments. Given the limited information that you have, you may have several tentative hypotheses (the number of spaces provided is not intended as a guide). What is the justification for each of the hypotheses? What further information would you require to confirm or reject each of these?

If you want to keep the book unmarked, use the photocopiable sheets on pp. 232–239.

JN's difficulties compromise the

Justification for this is that

JN's difficulties compromise the

Justification for this is that

JN's difficulties compromise the

Justification for this is that

JN's difficulties compromise the

Justification for this is that

What other factors need to be taken into consideration in planning assessments for JN?

Our hypotheses

> When you have completed your hypotheses, compare them to our suggestions. As you can see, it is not possible to propose firm hypotheses, but tentative possibilities can guide the selection of assessments, and each assessment should contribute to the identification of the level of deficit.

JN's difficulties compromise visual processing and this may interfere with all assessments which depend on visual input.

Justification for this is that on naming objects of pictures, her responses sometimes indicated that she did not recognise them and she made visual errors on the word–picture matching assessment.

JN's difficulties compromise auditory processing. Further assessment will be required to narrow down a more specific hypothesis. Distinction between impairments in auditory phonological analysis, in the phonological input lexicon or access to the semantic system is required.

Justification for this is that her relatives reported that they have to repeat themselves before she seems to understand what they are saying. A central semantic impairment or hearing loss could also account for this behaviour (see below).

JN's difficulties compromise the semantic system.

Justification for this is that JN appears to have comprehension difficulties with single words which affect both the input modalities of hearing and reading and the output modalities of speech and writing.

Other factors that need to be taken into consideration in planning assessment include the possibility that JN may have visuo-spatial as well as visual difficulties, as there is evidence from the CT scan of bilateral parieto-occipital lesions. Given her age, her previous employment in a sewing factory and her relatives' reports of her requiring repetition for understanding, possible hearing loss should also be considered. Finally, her relatives' reports of mild memory problems before her stroke and mild confusions since her return home, in the context of evidence of three infarcts identified at the later CT scan, suggest that JN may have a generalised cognitive deficit.

Your selection of assessments

Now that you have some initial hypotheses about the loci of impairments, plan the types of assessment tasks that you would employ to test out your hypotheses. We have provided spaces for several assessments, but this does not mean that we expect you to use the exact number. You will find that selection of one assessment will be influenced by the potential findings of previous ones carried out.

Assessment

Justification for selection

Assessment

Justification for selection

Assessment

Justification for selection

Assessment

Justification for selection

Assessment

Justification for selection

Assessment

Justification for selection

Our selection of assessments

> Now you have selected possible assessments compare them to the suggestions that we have made. Remember that there is no single right way of assessing someone using a psycholinguistic perspective. You should, however, be able to justify the need for each of the assessments in testing out specific hypotheses regarding the locus of impairment. If you selected different assessments, look at the assessments that were selected and work out the rationale behind them.

Assessment: A concept associative task using pictures, i.e. the *Pyramids and Palm Trees Test.*

Justification for selection: This will give some quantification of JN's ability to infer concepts from line drawings and make semantic links without the (overt) use of words. From her comments on the drawings, it will also give opportunities for any visual misrecognitions to be revealed. A comparison of the results with those from the reading version of this test would also be relevant, to allow a direct comparison of the effect of different modes of input on JN's semantic processing. Since the same items are used, it would be necessary to have an interval between the presentations.

Assessment: Audiometric screening test.

Justification for selection: A hearing test will allow identification of any peripheral hearing loss and indicate whether referral for a full audiometric examination should be considered. If JN does have a significant hearing loss, further assessment of auditory phonological processing and auditory lexical processing (see below) is not indicated, as performance on these assessments which require fine auditory discriminations would be predicted as poor on the basis of the hearing loss; thus it will not be possible to interpret performance in relation to language processing deficits.

Assessment: Auditory discrimination assessments. Possible assessments include PALPA 1 *Non-word minimal pairs*, PALPA 2 *Word minimal pairs*, PALPA 4 *Word minimal pairs requiring picture selection*, ADACB P1 *Non-word minimal pairs* and ADACB P3 *Real word minimal pairs*.

Justification for selection: These assessments will allow exploration of auditory phonological analysis. If JN is able to make the fine discriminations required by these assessments, it will allow us to rule out impairment in auditory phonological analysis as underlying her comprehension impairment. As noted above, these assessments would not be appropriate if JN was found to have significantly impaired hearing.

Assessment: Assessment of auditory lexical decision, for example, PALPA 5 *Auditory lexical decision: imageability × frequency* or ADACB L1 *Lexical decision test.*

Justification for selection: If JN's performance on the hearing test or auditory discrimination assessments is poor, it will not be necessary to undertake this assessment because it can be predicted that her performance will be poor on the basis of impaired hearing or auditory phonological analysis. If she performs well on these assessments, however, investigation of lexical decision will allow us to check whether she has impairment involving the phonological input lexicon.

Assessment: A test of semantic processing which does not use picture input. Possible assessments include PALPA 49 *Auditory synonym judgement*, PALPA 50 *Written synonym judgement*, ADACB S1 *Auditory synonym matching*, ADACB S1Wr *Written synonym judgement* and PALPA 51 *Word semantic association.*

Justification for selection: The use of semantic tasks which do not involve pictures will allow investigation of JN's semantic processing without visual processing deficits confounding performance. These assessments are all controlled for imageability and will therefore allow examination of the predicted influence of imageability often associated with a central semantic disorder. Comparison of performance on assessments in both spoken and written modality will allow exploration of how far the disorder is supramodal.

Assessment: A picture naming test, such as PALPA 54 *Picture naming × frequency* or the *Boston Naming Test.*

Justification for selection: This will give some measure of JN's lexical retrieval difficulties, although it will be necessary to consider any confounding effects of impairment to visual processing. Analysis of the pattern of performance should provide information to inform the hypotheses about the impairments underlying lexical retrieval deficits. With a central semantic disorder we would expect semantic paraphasias to be produced, with some failures to name and failure to recognise the correct word when it is offered to her.

Assessment: A test of writing, such as PALPA 40: *Imageability × frequency*.

Justification for selection: There is a suggestion that JN may have visuo-spatial difficulties, and if so this could impair her ability to write. A test of writing which is controlled for the semantic factor of imageability could give additional information on her semantic abilities as well as on other levels in the written production of words. If her hearing proves adequate, a task like PALPA 40 using dictation would avoid the possible difficulties in using pictures as is required in written picture naming.

Assessment results

> Now read through the results of the assessments that we actually carried out.

Pyramids and Palm Trees Test (picture version)

JN obtained a score of 46 out of 52, showing a moderate degree of impairment. Two misrecognitions were recorded. The reading version of this assessment was not undertaken.

Audiometric screening test

A screening pure-tone test showed a 40 dB loss in both ears. Since this is not a severe loss in someone of JN's age, it was decided to proceed with the auditory tests.

PALPA 1 Non-word minimal pairs

JN's scores revealed impairment but were above chance at 71%. She scored 27/36 for pairs which were different. There was no effect of position or type of articulatory contrast.

PALPA 5 Auditory lexical decision

JN's scored 53/80 on this assessment, performing at chance on low imageability items.

PALPA 49 Auditory synonym judgement

JN scored 35 out of 60 on this assessment, with poorer performance for low-imageability pairs and more errors in rejecting synonyms than non-synonyms as shown below:

Synonym pairs: High-imageability, 6 out of 15
                    Low-imageability, 3 out of 15
Non-synonym pairs   High-imageability 10 out of 15
                    Low-imageability, 6 out of 15

PALPA 51 Word semantic association

JN was impaired on this assessment (which uses reading) for both high- and low-imageability items, but with a particularly poor performance for the low imageability items:

High-imageability   9 out of 15 (4 semantic errors, 2 unrelated errors)
Low-imageability   1 out of 15 (6 semantic errors, 8 unrelated errors)

Boston Naming Test

JN scored 30 out of 60 on this assessment with the following error pattern:

- thirteen no responses (e.g. 'don't know what that is', 'no I couldn't say that')
- seven semantic paraphasias (e.g. 'ladder' for stilts, 'plant' for cactus, 'tape measure' for protractor)
- six phonological/ verbal paraphasias (e.g. 'rhododendron' for rhinoceros, 'a tri something' for tripod)
- four visual misrecognitions (e.g. hammock described as 'like a little ironing board'; compass 'I think there's a bird on there'; pyramid 'it's like an animal, I'm not sure, it might be a little bit like a tent'; stethoscope 'is that a brush?').

Several responses contained personalised comments (e.g. 'I used to have a door like that') and other circumlocutions (e.g. 'people saying something' for scroll). When given the target by the therapist, she rejected it on four occasions. Phonemic cues were successful on three occasions.

PALPA 40 Imageability × frequency spelling

JN achieved 8/40 on this test, including two self-corrections. Five of her correct items were HIHF, with one each in the other categories of HILF, LIHF and LILF. Most of her errors were neologisms (e.g. *volate* for valour). She made three (probable) semantic paragraphias (*Flame* for fire, *Tomatioes* for tobacco, *Flue* for funnel). She made three partial perseverations: after writing *summer* correctly, she wrote *sumer* for thing and *simmer for* coffee, and, after writing *Rowel* for wrath, *grovel* for gravy. She used the correct initial letter for 35 out of the 40 words, and showed knowledge of the correct number of syllables (though not necessarily letters) for 31 words e.g. *spitich* for spider, *bonish* for bonus. Some errors were only of single letter substitutions e.g. *slove* for slope, and *attifude*.

Your interpretation of the results of the assessments

What do the assessment results mean? Map out your hypotheses of the locus or loci of JN's impairment, using the diagram of the model. Indicate also what processes seem to be preserved and which levels you are uncertain about from the assessment results so far. Note down the justification in support of your hypotheses.

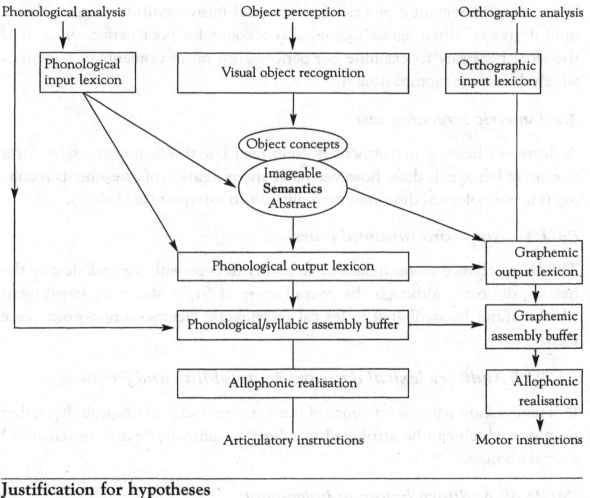

Justification for hypotheses

Our interpretation of the results of the assessments

> Now read through our interpretation of the psycholinguistic findings.

Pyramids and Palm Trees Test

JN's performance on this assessment was impaired. Although this may reflect an impairment in semantic processing, her visual misrecognitions suggest that a mild degree of visual agnosia could also account for poor performance. It is therefore necessary to examine her performance on assessments of semantics which do not use picture stimuli.

Audiometric screening test

A degree of hearing impairment is confirmed but this is not excessive for a woman of her age. It does, however, make interpretation of assessments requiring fine phonological discrimination difficult to interpret (see below).

PALPA 1 Non-word minimal pairs

The above-chance scores indicated an ability to cope with the task despite the hearing difficulty, although the overall score of 51/72 shows an impairment which cannot be attributed to lexical or semantic factors, as non-words were used.

PALPA 5 Auditory lexical decision: imageability and frequency

JN's results show a major influence of the semantic factor of imageability, rather than one which can be attributed to a hearing difficulty or a (non-semantic) lexical disorder.

PALPA 49 Auditory synonym judgement

JN's overall score at 25 out of 60 is at chance. Although it is possible that impaired hearing, impaired auditory processing or impaired ability to hold two items in auditory short-term memory underly this performance, the better performance for high imageability items supports the hypothesis of either a central semantic impairment or impaired access to the semantic system from the phonological input lexicon.

PALPA 51 Word semantic association

As JN performed poorly on this semantic assessment, which uses access from reading, and also shows an effect of imageability, it is probable that the impairment is a central one, rather than solely in access from either modality. This is further supported by her picture-naming performance (see below). The occurrence of unrelated errors may, however, indicate concomitant impairment in orthographic analysis, the orthographic input lexicon or in access to the semantic system from the lexicon.

Boston Naming Test

Her overall score indicates a severe degree of anomia. The types of errors she makes are consistent with the hypothesis that she has a central semantic disorder, i.e. the number of uncorrected semantic paraphasias and no responses and her rejections of the correct word when given by the examiner. As all these items are highly imageable, the central semantic disorder does not seem to be restricted to low imageable items. She is sometimes able to access partial phonological information about items she does not retrieve (the phonological/verbal paraphasias) and is occasionally helped by a phonemic or syllabic cue. There is further confirmation that she has some problems in visual recognition of drawings.

PALPA 40 Imageability × frequency spelling

There was no sign of visuo-spatial problems in JN's writing to dictation. Her semantic difficulties showed in the semantic paragraphias and in the influence of imageability (6 HI correct, 2LI correct), although it should be noted that imageability influenced the results from the PALPA controls. Her perseverations towards the end of the first half of the list probably indicate a build-up of fatigue. Her knowledge of the first letter and number of syllables suggests that the phonological representation of the words gave better access to the graphemic lexicon than she received from semantics (e.g. in writing *trasing* for treason).

Conversation analysis: selecting parameters for assessment

> We will ask you shortly what inferences for therapy you might draw from the psycholinguistic findings. Meanwhile from the results of the cognitive neuropsychological assessment and the information given in the case description, consider what analyses of conversation you would like to undertake to gain information to guide therapy.

Conversational data to be collected

_____

_____

Analysis

_____

Justification for selection

_____

_____

_____

_____

_____

_____

Analysis

_____

Justification for selection

_____

_____

_____

_____

_____

_____

Analysis

Justification for selection

Justification for selection: The cognitive neuropsychological assessments have identified a central semantic impairment which compromise comprehension and results in anomia. In addition, JN has impaired articulation and other possible impairments in auditory processing which compromise auditory comprehension. Examination of the manifestation of these in conversation and analysis of how JN and her interlocutors deal with them will therefore be useful. It may be possible to more successful strategy's which are being used in collaboration, and encourage the development of these in therapy.

Our selection of parameters for conversation analysis

> Now that you have selected some possible analyses, compare them to the suggestions that we have made. If you selected different analyses, look at the ones that we selected and work out the rationale behind this choice.

Conversational data to be collected: JN's most frequent conversational partner is her sister, who lives nearby, and, to a less extent, her daughter who is at work all day. As JN tires during the course of the day, a recording of conversation between her and her sister made at home during the early afternoon would seem to be the most appropriate.

Analysis: Repair patterns.

Justification for selection: The cognitive neuropsychological assessments have identified a central semantic impairment which compromises comprehension and results in anomia. In addition, JN has impaired hearing and other possible impairments in auditory processing which compromise auditory comprehension. Examination of the manifestation of these in conversation and analysis of how JN and her interlocutors deal with them will therefore be useful. It may be possible to note successful strategies which are being used in collaborative repairs, and encourage the development of these in therapy.

Analysis: Topic management.

Justification for selection: As JN has been described as being occasionally confused and forgetful, she may have some difficulties with topic initiation or maintenance, or in avoiding topic repetitions. A number of personalisations were noted in her responses to the Boston Naming Test, and these may indicate that she may have difficulties in maintaining topics which are not personally directed.

Analysis: Turn-taking.

Justification for selection: JN's performance on the picture-naming assessment identified that she sometimes fails to retrieve words. This impairment may influence her ability to take a turn in conversation without a delay and to complete her turns. Examination of whether word retrieval failures occur in conversation and how these impact on turn-taking would therefore be worth examining.

Results of the conversation analyses

> Now read through the findings of the analyses undertaken.

Conversational data collected: A recording was made at JN's home of a conversation between her and her sister. A radiomicrophone was available at this time, which enabled the recordings to be made without restriction of movement and by the sister without anyone else being present.

Analysis of repair patterns: Manifestations of JN's semantic processing impairment could be identified in the conversation with her sister. JN produced identifiable uncorrected semantic errors. These did not, however, become the focus of repair work because her sister was able to use the context to understand the target that JN intended, for example in the production of 'strong' for 'big' in the following excerpt in which JN and her sister are talking about a dishcloth that JN is crocheting:

1. JN   that too strong for you?
2. CP   no that's big enough
3. JN   well you can have that one (5 syll.)
4. CP   what do you think?
5. JN   yeah I thought it was a bit big but you thought no

Her sister is able to produce a response to JN's question despite the semantic paraphasia. Within her turn, she embeds a correction of the paraphasia and the topic develops without the need for repair work.

A further manifestation of JN's semantic impairment observed in the conversation was the use of pronouns and proforms to refer. There were several repair sequences in which her sister asked for clarification of a vague referent. Approximately half of these were quickly resolved, with JN's sister asking for clarification and JN providing it. For the other half, resolution was not achieved, as seen in the following extract in which JN had initiated T1 after a 17-second lapse in the conversation:

1. JN   she's coming to see us anyway
2. CP   hmmm?

3. JN   she's coming to see us
4. CP   who, Jennifer?
5. JN   no
         (5.5)
6. JN   they heavy for me I don't know what

JN's sister initiated clarification with 'hmmm?' in T2. JN treated this as a hearing check and repeated her previous turn. Her sister responded to this by asking for more explicit clarification and putting forward a candidate referent for 'she'. JN rejected this but did no further clarification work herself. Following a 5.5-second silence, a new topic was initiated.

In addition to repair sequences being initiated for clarification on specific referents, on a number of occasions JN produced long turns, on which her sister asked for some general clarification, as seen in the following extract:

1. JN   and she says I I was sleeping with her
         (2.0)
2. JN   I a sleeping with with somewhere I don't know
         (2.0)
3. JN   and she says eee Jenny she says I felt terribly (2 syll.) so I says why you
         can post post me
4.   (3.0)
5. JN   so she said oh well that'll be alright I'll post to you
         (2.5)
6. JN   I'll just post you one
         (1.0)
7. CP   is that when she went to Blyth?
8. JN   when Jennifer took her <mmhm>
9. JN   <took her> yes

In this extract JN produced a narrative about a mutual acquaintance. Her sister did not initiate repair work on any part of it but allowed JN to continue until in T7 she asks for clarification about when the event that JN is talking about happened. While to the naive listener, it is difficult to interpret JN's T1–6, it appears that JN's sister with her shared knowledge was able to follow her.

No manifestations of JN's impaired auditory comprehension or hearing were identified in the conversation. JN initiated no repair sequences on her conversational partner's turns to seek clarification and there were no occurrences of repair sequences arising as a consequence of JN misunderstanding or mishearing one of her conversational partner's turns.

Analysis of topic management: JN and her sister participated equally in topic initiation. JN initiated five topics (dishcloth, heating, Christmas cards, Christmas shop window displays and her daughter's visit), while her sister initiated four (Christmas lights, a friend's telephone call, dishcloths again, passer-by seen through the window). JN maintained the topics through several turns, and showed no tendency to repeat topics.

Analysis of turn-taking: In contrast to the word-finding failures in the psycholinguistic assessments, there were very few pauses arising as a consequence of failures in word finding. Instead, JN tended to produce either pronouns or to omit words and continue with a further utterance as in the following example:

JN   Eee if I were a (0.5) I would I would wrote some Christmas cards

Where within-pauses did occur, JN's sister tolerated them and did not use them to take the conversational floor.

Planning initial intervention

From the findings of these assessment results it is proposed that JN has a central semantic impairment which underlies her lexical retrieval deficits and her difficulties in auditory comprehension. She may also have impairment in auditory processing, although her hearing loss makes it difficult to establish this. Conversation analysis indicates that JN nevertheless participates relatively effectively in communication in a one-to-one domestic situation with a familiar partner. What therapy would you derive from the findings of the psycholinguistic assessments and the conversation analysis?

Our suggestions for initial intervention

> Now that you have thought about some possible interventions, compare them with our suggestions. Remember that these are only tentative ideas and may differ from yours. Both your and our ideas may be appropriate. The important issue is that intervention should be motivated by theoretical principles.

The main deficit identified from the psycholinguistic assessments was a central semantic impairment. This had an impact on conversation in relation to JN's word finding, although interestingly, in the conversation, there was no evidence that it gave rise to breakdowns in comprehension, suggesting that enough context is provided in conversation (at least with a highly familiar conversational partner) to compensate for the semantic impairment.

Impairment-focused intervention using a semantic therapy programme could be attempted to remediate JN's central semantic impairment. There are numerous approaches commonly used to treat semantic impairments. These include semantic categorisation tasks, word–picture matching with distractors of increasingly close semantic relationship and selecting items to definitions. Studies of semantic therapy are outlined in our suggestions for initial intervention with Case 1, Mr AR.

Because JN has greater difficulty in understanding low-imageability words, it would be appropriate to begin with high-imageability words, perhaps reducing JN's occasional problems with visual recognition by using coloured photographs rather than line drawings. There is some controversy as to whether abstract (or low-imageability) words form a separate semantic category (see Franklin, Howard and Patterson, 1995), and at this stage it may not be desirable to attempt to extend the semantic therapy to low-imageability words.

As JN has supramodal difficulties in semantics, use of non-speech modalities (reading, writing, spelling, gesturing, drawing) would not be expected to be of major assistance in facilitating communication during collaborative repairs. In view of JN's bilateral brain damage and her occasional confusions, as well as in the light of her relatively good communicative functioning, it would be particularly important not to put her under undue stress, nor to persist in direct therapy unless an evaluation confirmed that it was having an effect on semantic processing.

JN should be consulted as to whether she wishes to be referred for a full audiometric investigation. It may be sufficient for her family to be advised to encourage lip-reading, minimise background noise and ensure JN's placement where she can hear best. The conversation analysis indicates that, at least in dyadic conversations, impaired hearing is not causing interactional difficulty.

JN is an equal participant in conversation, introduces and maintains topics adequately, and has her share of turns in conversation with her sister, who is tolerant of the few within-turn delays that JN produces. In the conversation, her sister demonstrates effective strategies to deal with semantic errors and vague referents. The high level of shared knowledge that exists between them contributes to this. JN does not show awareness of the semantic errors or problematic non-specific referring expressions that she uses, as there are no self-repair attempts. It may be a fruitful therapy approach to combine direct work on semantic processing with work on strategies for JN and her sister. This could include reinforcement and development of the effective strategies that JN's sister is already using. Resolution of repair may be improved by it being made explicit exactly what the problem with her conversational turn is, for example, the use of wh- questions for clarification rather than general repair initiators like 'hmm?', which she frequently uses. In addition, work with JN to recognise precisely the type of clarification that her sister needs may be useful.

Both her relatives have expressed the desire to know more about JN's aphasia, and it would be appropriate to supply them with a personalised booklet explaining what a stroke is, what language processes may be disturbed and what JN's particular problems are. Material for such booklets is available from Action for Dysphasic Adults (York Cognitive Neuropsychological Research Group, 1996). Advice on conversational management could also be incorporated, using specific illustrations from the transcripts of the recordings (Lesser and Algar, 1995; Booth and Perkins, 1999).

In view of JN's sociability and good mobility, and the fact that she is living on her own, it may be appropriate to ask her if she would wish to attend a Speech-after-Stroke Club, if a suitable one is available.

Developing the hypotheses

> Remember that the results of assessment (and of intervention) feed back into developing the hypotheses you initially made. There may also be gaps in your interpretation, which the results have revealed. Use this page to write down what further investigations you might wish to consider to develop your hypotheses, some of which may depend on JN's response to therapy. **Cover up the next page (which has our suggestions) until you have written yours down.**

Our suggestions for developing the hypotheses

> Now read through the suggestions that we have made and compare them with your own.

Although JN's severe semantic deficit has not impeded her ability to participate in the conversation with her sister due to the knowledge which they share, it would be desirable to assess how she might cope with less familiar partners. This would be particularly relevant if she were to wish to join a Speech-after-Stroke Club. A recording could therefore be made of a conversation between JN and her daughter, or a less familiar visitor, such as a student therapist. An assessment such as CAPPA (Whitworth, Perkins and Lesser, 1997) would permit a comparison to be made between conversational behaviours as reported by JN's sister or daughter, and those in the actual sample of conversation obtained. The CAPPA interview could also help to establish the degree of concern the relative experiences about what the therapist considers to be JN's problems in communication. It would also give further information on the strategies used by the conversationalists to accommodate to these problems. A section of CAPPA also seeks information on pre-morbid styles and on whether opportunities for interaction have been reduced following the onset of aphasia.

There are also other aspects of psycholinguistic processing which could be considered. The results of PALPA 51 *Word semantic association* suggested the possibility of some specific impairments in reading. This could be further investigated through the range of reading tests in PALPA 19 to 27 and PALPA 31, in order to explore whether an additional (non-semantic) deficit might lie in orthographic analysis or the orthographic input lexicon. Comparison could also be made of word-retrieval in different semantic categories. Another aspect is the comprehension of sentences. A preliminary assessment to explore this could be the Test for the Reception of Grammar (TROG) (Bishop, 1983), used with care, in view of JN's visual difficulties.

As JN was reported to have made an error in selecting a £10 note, her ability to manipulate numbers and perform calculations, such as are needed for shopping, could be investigated (Christensen, 1974, Section L))

In view of JN's bilateral parieto-occipital infarcts, she could be screened for cognitive dysfunctions, which have been linked in some cases to right hemisphere or bilateral damage. One of these is impaired appreciation of humour and metaphor (see Bryan's Right Hemisphere Battery, 1989). JN's difficulties in recognising pictures may also be associated with other problems in visuo-spatial recognition, which could be explored through the Visual Object and Space Perception Battery (VOSP) (Warrington and James, 1991), or parts of the Rivermead Perceptual Assessment Battery (RPAB) (Whiting et al., 1985, Tests 13 and 14)

In view of JN's reported memory impairment, if this appears to increase in severity, there are a number of measures, such as the Rivermead Behavioural Memory Test (RBMT) (Wilson, Cockburn and Baddeley, 1985, currently under revision) or the Autobiographical Memory Interview (Kopelman, Wilson and Baddeley, 1990), which could be used to quantify this for future monitoring in association with a clinical psychologist. A test of everyday attention, such as Robertson et al.'s (1994) test of that name, would also help to give quantified information on the extent to which her confusions were affecting everyday life. It would, however, be very important not to overload JN with formal assessments. The suggestions above have been listed as examples of aspects of cognition which could be examined in more detail, if the interactions between the therapist and JN or her relatives suggest that they may be having an impact on JN's everyday life. Should such a potential deterioration happen, a referral for further investigation would be appropriate.

Case 6
Mr AC

When you work through this case remember to read the information first and then write down your own interpretation and ideas before you turn the page to read ours.

Initial impressions

> Read through the case description and think about what the important features are that will guide your selection of assessments.

Case description

AC is a 69-year-old retired police officer who lives with his wife. They have two daughters, a son and a number of grandchildren, all of whom live nearby and whom they see regularly. His most frequent visitor is his younger daughter who has a part-time job at the local community college and who visits her parents three or four times a week.

AC had received 9 years of formal education, and after this had taken a number of correspondence courses relating to his profession.

A left cerebral stroke left AC with jargon speech and problems in comprehension. He did not lose consciousness at the onset of the CVA and was not hemiplegic. As a consequence he was not admitted to hospital. Five months later, as his speech and language difficulties had not cleared up, his GP referred him for speech and language therapy.

AC complained of difficulty in both following conversation and following programmes on the television. His wife commented that he frequently requested repetitions, although both reported that his hearing has always been very good.

On PALPA 53 *Spoken picture naming* he named 35 out of 40 items correctly, although for several items he had a long response latency. He made three semantic errors, two phonemic paraphasias which he attempted to correct, for the items 'elephant' and 'lemon'. He also produced phonemic paraphasias and demonstrated mild word-finding difficulties in his spontaneous speech, as illustrated in the following extract from conversation with the therapist:

CP   and that's where you think you picked up the meningitis?
AC   well I'm thinking that's where it got from them but the thing about it was that they took the well after I'd pulled myself round a bit they put me back into the er (1:2) hospitals and [ɛʔɛlɪvəns] where you get your [ɛlɪvəns] or you get you (1:0) hhh er:: (1:6) [kalf kəl kʊlvənəns kʊlf kə]
CP   convalescence?

AC was a keen reader before he had his stroke but has now reported that he finds reading difficult.

Your initial hypotheses

> Using the information given in the case description, consider the possible loci of AC's impairments. Given the limited information that you have, you may have several tentative hypotheses (the number of spaces provided is not intended as a guide). What is the justification for each of the hypotheses? What further information would you require to confirm or reject each of these?

If you want to keep the book unmarked, use the photocopiable sheets on pp. 232–239.

AC's difficulties compromise the

Justification for this is that

AC's difficulties compromise the

Justification for this is that

AC's difficulties compromise the

Justification for this is that

AC's difficulties compromise the

Justification for this is that

AC's difficulties compromise the

Justification for this is that

What other factors need to be taken into consideration in planning assessments for AC?

Our hypotheses

> When you have completed your hypotheses, compare them to our suggestions. As you can see, it is not possible to propose firm hypotheses, but tentative possibilities can guide the selection of assessments, and each assessment should contribute to the identification of the level of deficit.

AC's difficulties compromise auditory phonological analysis.

Justification for this is that he reports comprehension difficulties in conversation. Although this may arise from impaired processing at a number of different levels (see below), his requests for repetitions in the light of good hearing may indicate a problem at this level.

AC's difficulties compromise the phonological input lexicon.

Justification for this is that he is reporting comprehension difficulties in conversation. Although, as noted above, there are a number of potential loci which could account for this deficit, if phonological analysis is intact, a deficit in the phonological input lexicon could potentially explain his comprehension deficit.

AC's difficulties compromise the semantic system.

Justification for this is that he produced semantic errors on the picture-naming assessment. While semantic errors in production can arise from impaired access to the phonological output lexicon (see below), it is possible that a central semantic impairment underlies these errors and the comprehension problems that he is reporting.

AC's difficulties compromise the phonological output lexicon.

Justification for this is that he showed a latency on the picture-naming test. The items on this test are all of relatively high frequency and he may experience greater difficulty for low-frequency words. An impairment in access to the phonological output lexicon could also account for the semantic paraphasias he produces, as well as for the delays in his naming.

AC's difficulties compromise the phonological assembly buffer.

Justification for this is that he produces phonemic paraphasias both on the naming test and in conversation. He appears to have particular difficulty with longer words. He produced phonological errors on two- and three-syllable words in PALPA 53 *Spoken picture naming*, but did not make this type of error on the majority of items which are only one syllable. An effect of syllable length is consistent with impairment to the assembly buffer.

Other factors that need to be taken into consideration in planning assessments include AC's comprehension deficit, which may interfere with his ability to follow task instructions. It will also be important to find out more about the severity of his reading difficulties if assessments which include the use of reading are to be employed.

Your selection of assessments

Now that you have some initial hypotheses about the loci of impairments, plan the types of assessment tasks that you would employ to test out your hypotheses. We have provided spaces for several assessments, but this does not mean that we expect you to use the exact number. You will find that selection of one assessment will be influenced by the potential findings of previous ones carried out.

Assessment

Justification for selection

Assessment

Justification for selection

Assessment

Justification for selection

Assessment

Justification for selection

Assessment

Justification for selection

Our selection of assessments

Now you have selected possible assessments compare them to the suggestions that we have made. Remember that there is no single right way of assessing someone using a psycholinguistic perspective. You should, however, be able to justify the need for each of the assessments in testing out specific hypotheses regarding the locus of impairment. If you selected different assessments, look at the assessments that were selected and work out the rationale behind this choice.

Assessment: Auditory discrimination assessments. Possible assessments include PALPA 1 *Non-word minimal pairs*, PALPA 2 *Word minimal pairs*, ADACB P1 *Non-word minimal pairs* and ADACB P3 *Real word minimal pairs*. PALPA 3 *Word minimal pairs requiring written selection* could be used if AC's reading ability is not too compromised.

Justification for selection: Results on these tests should help to give information on AC's processing abilities at the level of phonological analysis. If AC performs well in the discrimination tasks this will provide support to his report of good hearing.

Assessment: Assessment of auditory lexical decision, for example, PALPA 5 *Auditory lexical decision: imageability × frequency* or ADACB L1 *Lexical decision*.

Justification for selection: If AC's performance on auditory discrimination assessments is poor, it will not be necessary to undertake this assessment as it can be predicted that his performance will be poor on the basis of impaired auditory phonological analysis. If he performs well on these assessments, however, investigation of lexical decision will allow us to check whether he has impairment involving the phonological input lexicon.

Assessment: Assessment of semantic processing using different input modalities. Possible assessments include PALPA 47 *Spoken word–picture matching* and PALPA 48 *Written word–picture matching* or ADACB S2 *Auditory word–picture matching* and ADACB S2Wr *Written word–picture matching*. If performance on assessments of this type were to be good, assessments that explored semantics for low-imageability items could be used. Suitable assessments for this would include PALPA 49 *Auditory synonym judgement* and PALPA 50 *Written synonym judgement* or ADACB S1 *Auditory synonym judgement* and ADACB S1Wr *Written synonym judgement*.

Justification for selection: These tests should provide some evidence relevant to the hypothesis that AC has a central semantic disorder. The word–picture tests include semantic distractors, which may tax him, and the synonym judgement tests allow for a comparison between high- and low-imageability items, which may throw some light on the nature of any semantic disorder. Comparison of performance across auditory and written versions of assessments will allow examination of whether AC has a central semantic impairment or impaired access to the semantic system.

Assessment: A picture-naming assessment which controls for word length and word frequency, such as the Mono-poly Naming Test .

Justification for selection: This naming assessment will allow further exploration of AC's difficulties in word production. An effect of the number of syllables in the word with a phonological error pattern would support the hypothesis that he has an impairment involving the phonological assembly buffer. The much lower-frequency items for this assessment in comparison to PALPA 53 *Spoken picture naming* will identify whether word frequency influences word retrieval ability. Poorer performance with lower-frequency items may indicate impairment involving the phonological output lexicon.

Assessment: A repetition assessment. A number of different variables could be examined. Possible assessments include PALPA 8 *Repetition of non-words*, PALPA 9 *Repetition of words: frequency × imageability*, ADACB L2 *Repetition of words* and repetition (on a different assessment occasion) of the words in the Mono-poly Picture Naming Test

Justification for selection: Repetition will allow examination of AC's phonological output processing, without requiring him to search for the lexical form of the word. If the hypothesis that AC has an impairment involving the phonological assembly buffer is correct, impaired repetition on all of these tasks with a phonological error pattern and deterioration in performance with increasing word length would be expected. With a 'pure' assembly disorder, it would be hypothesised that there would be no effect of imageability or word frequency; in fact AC should perform as well (or as badly) on non-words as words. If he has an impairment in phonological analysis, this would impair repetition ability. It will therefore be necessary to interpret his performance on repetition in the light of his performance on auditory discrimination assessments (see above).

Assessment: An oral reading assessment. Possibilies include PALPA 31 *Oral reading: imageability × frequency*, which uses the same items as PALPA 9 *Repetition of words* or reading (on a different assessment occasion) of the words in the Mono-poly Naming Test.

Justification for selection: Oral reading would allow examination of AC's output difficulties with different input from naming or repetition. As for repetition, if the hypothesis that AC has an impairment involving the phonological assembly buffer is correct, impaired oral reading with a phonological error pattern and deterioration in performance with increasing word length would be expected. With a 'pure' assembly disorder, it would be hypothesised that there would be no effect of imageability or word frequency. It would be important to analyse his error pattern carefully, as we have no information about whether orthographic input processing is intact and this may affect his performance.

Assessment results

Now read through the results of the assessments that we actually carried out.

PALPA 1 Non-word minimal pairs

AC scored 67 out of 72, which is within the range of the PALPA control subjects.

PALPA 5 Auditory lexical decision: imageability × frequency

AC scored 155 out of 160 on auditory lexical decision, which is within the range of the PALPA control subjects.

PALPA 47 Spoken word–picture matching and PALPA 48 Written word–picture matching

AC achieved maximum scores on word–picture matching in both the auditory and written versions, i.e. 40 out of 40.

PALPA 49 Auditory synonym judgement and PALPA 50 Written synonym judgement

On the auditory version AC was impaired, scoring 50 out of 60 with seven errors for low-imageability items and three errors for high-imageability items. He found the task difficult and frequently asked for repetition of items. Performance on the written version of this task was much more rapid. He scored 58 out of 60, which is within the normal range of the PALPA control subjects.

Mono-poly Naming Test

As some of AC's productions showed extended phonological searching behaviours, this test was scored in two ways, i.e. for correct names produced within 5 seconds, and for correct names produced despite longer delays. AC's score within the 5-second measure was 36 out of 60, comprising 23 out of 30 mono-syllabic words and 13 out of 30 polysyllabic words. Inclusion of the names produced after 5 seconds increased these scores to 27 out of 30 and 21 out of 30 respectively. The pattern of errors included six phonemic paraphasias, two neologisms and four failures to name. Responses frequently involved multiple phonological attempts at the target (conduit d'approche), as seen in the following example:

> 'dominoes' -> [mɛʔ mɛʔ mɛʔ 'mɛnədops] the dice (4.0) [pɛl] what do you [pɛl] dice (4.0) oh dear dear this here (4.0) ["dɛmi] dominoes.

There were also a few examples where delayed correct responses appeared to arise from an initial failure to retrieve the lexical item, as illustrated in the following example:

> 'envelope' -> (3.0) post (1.0) letter post (2.0) envelope.

In some cases all the phonemes of the target word were present but were misordered, with AC uncertain as to whether he had produced the correct form, for example:

> 'unicorn' -> [s:] yes [skə 'skɔnijən 'skɔnijən] (5.0) erm [skə] (2.0) ['kɔnijən 'kɔnij ən 'kɔnijən] I don't know whether that's right.

He produced the target response for 16 out of 20 of the higher-frequency items, 9 out of 20 of the medium-frequency items and 11 out of 20 of the low-frequency items.

PALPA 8 Repetition of non-words and PALPA 9 Repetition of words: frequency × imageability

On the tests of repetition AC was impaired with both non-words and words. His score on non-word repetition was 47 out of 80, with 26 of the errors being phonemic paraphasias, two neologistic productions and five real words. In all cases he maintained the correct number of syllables. His score on repetition of words was 61 out of 80, with a similar pattern of errors, i.e.12 phonemic paraphasias, two neologistic productions and five verbal paraphasias, such as 'value' for 'valour'. There was an effect of frequency (35 out of 40 on high-frequency items; 26 out of 40 on low-frequency items) and a smaller effect of imageability (34 out of 40 on high-imageability items; 27 out of 40 on low-imageability items).

PALPA 31 Oral reading: imageability × frequency

AC scored 75 out of 80 on this assessment, with correct responses produced without delay or revision. The five errors were phonemic paraphasias, all of which were self-corrected immediately. For example:

'treason' -> ['tɹisən 'tɹizən]
'gravity' -> ['gɹɛvəti 'gɹɛɪvəti 'gɹɛavəti]

There were no effects of frequency or imageability.

Your interpretation of the results of the assessments

> What do the assessment results mean? Map out your hypotheses of the locus or loci of AC's impairment, using the diagram of the model. Indicate also what processes seem to be preserved and which levels you are uncertain about from the assessment results so far. Note down the justification in support of your hypotheses.

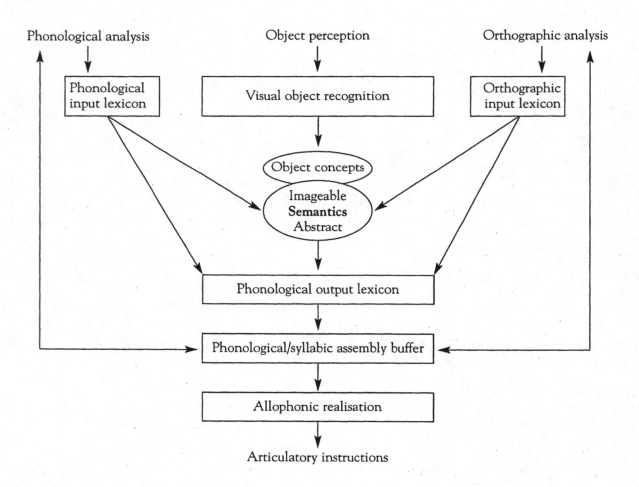

Justification for hypotheses

Our interpretation of the results of the assessments

> Now read through our interpretation of the psycholinguistic findings.

PALPA 1 Non-word minimal pairs

AC's performance within the normal range on this assessment indicates that he is not impaired in auditory phonological analysis. The results also indicate that he does not have a significant hearing loss.

PALPA 5 Auditory lexical decision: imageability × frequency

AC's performance within the normal range on this assessment suggests that processing at the level of the phonological input lexicon is not impaired.

PALPA 47 Spoken word–picture matching and PALPA 48 Written word–picture matching

AC's errorless performance in these assessments provides evidence that central semantic processing for at least high-imageability words is intact. This suggests that the small number of semantic errors that he makes arise from impaired access to the phonological output lexicon, with a lexical form of a semantic associate occasionally being accessed when activation for the target does not reach a threshold to achieve retrieval.

PALPA 49 Auditory synonym judgement and PALPA 50 Written synonym judgement

AC's performance on the written version of this assessment provides further evidence for intact central semantic processing. His impaired performance on the auditory test suggests that he may have an impairment in access to the semantic system from an intact phonological input lexicon. This appears to be a mild disorder, as he did not make a large number of errors. The marginally greater number of errors on low-imageability items may indicate that access is more impaired for low-imageability items, although with the small number of errors made this is not a clear pattern. An alternative explanation for AC's poorer performance on the auditory version is that he has a reduced auditory verbal memory span, which compromises the ability to hold two items in memory while making a judgement. He did, however, perform well on PALPA 1

Non-word minimal pairs, which requires judgement about two items presented in the auditory modality.

Mono-poly Naming Test

AC's performance on the naming test is consistent with compromised processing of the phonological assembly buffer. This is indicated by the multiple target-related phonological error pattern and the effect of number of syllables on his performance. Impairment at this level of processing would be predicted to have an effect on all word production, whatever the mode of output, and further evidence for an impairment at this level is provided by his performance on the repetition and oral reading assessments (see below).

Certain aspects of AC's performance on naming are consistent with some involvement of an impaired phonological output lexicon. First he showed an effect of word frequency. Second, for a number of items for which he produced a delayed correct response or a failed response, he showed no phonological knowledge of the target, despite often demonstrating semantic knowledge through rejected semantic paraphasias and circumlocutions. Thus for some items there appeared to be a failure to achieve sufficient activation in the phonological output lexicon to make an attempt at the target.

PALPA 8 Repetition of non-words and PALPA 9 Repetition of words: frequency × imageability

A's performance on the repetition tasks supports the hypothesis of an impairment at the level of the phonological assembly buffer. This is indicated by the phonological nature of the errors and the influence of number of syllables to be produced. AC was significantly better at repeating words than non-words, and this suggests that activation from the lexical routes must support performance. Evidence for this is the effect of frequency noted, suggesting that the phonological output lexicon is influencing the results, with some reduction of availability of less frequent words. The non-lexical route, however, must also be functioning to a degree, as he was able to repeat a proportion of non-words correctly.

PALPA 31 Oral reading: imageability × frequency

This assessment uses the same words as PALPA 8. The marked input modality difference with reading superior to repetition may arise from the fact that reading allows AC to refresh the assembly buffer with a continuous input, which is not available when he has only the auditory image of the word. Although the number of errors was reduced in reading, the quality of the errors was the same as that produced during the repetition task. An alternative explanation, keeping within the description given in the psycholinguistic model, would be of differentially impaired access to the phonological assembly buffer from the different processing routes involved in reading and repetition.

AC did not produce regularisation errors in oral reading, indicating that this input allows him to achieve enough access in the phonological output lexicon to retrieve the lexical form, in contrast to greater difficulty in oral naming where input to the lexicon only comes from the semantic system.

Conversation analysis: selecting parameters for assessment

> We will ask you shortly what inferences for therapy you might draw from the psycholinguistic findings. Meanwhile from the results of the cognitive neuropsychological assessment and the information given in the case description, consider what analyses of conversation you would like to undertake to gain information to guide therapy.

Conversational data to be collected

Analysis

Justification for selection

Analysis

Justification for selection

Analysis

Justification for selection

Our selection of parameters for conversation analysis

> Now that you have selected some possible analyses, compare them to the suggestions that we have made. If you selected different analyses, look at the ones that we selected and work out the rationale behind this choice.

Conversational data to be collected: As AC lives with his wife, initially a recording of a conversation with her was thought to be the most useful, in terms of informing intervention. Through discussion with AC and his wife about the purpose of assessment, however, a recording with his younger daughter was agreed upon. This was because AC reported that he and his wife had very little difficulty as they were always talking about everyday issues for which they had a high level of shared knowledge. AC reported that he experienced greater difficulty in conversations with other family members and friends.

Analysis: Repair patterns.

Justification for selection: As AC makes a large number of phonemic paraphasias and experiences some difficulties in lexical retrieval on formal tasks, it will be expected that he and his partner will engage in a number of repair activities. In particular his repair strategies can be analysed according to how successful he is at self-repairing errors, given the multiple revision attempts seen in his performance on oral picture naming. Examination of how AC and his daughter handle trouble sources which AC cannot resolve himself through collaborative repair will be informative. Although on single-word processing assessments, only very mild deficits in auditory comprehension were identified, as AC reports functional difficulties in this area, identification of trouble sources arising from breakdowns in comprehension should be sought and an examination made of the strategies that the conversationalists use to deal with them.

Analysis: Turn-taking.

Justification for selection: As AC shows occasional retrieval problems from the phonological output lexicon, apparently independently of his phonological assembly difficulties, there may be delays before he takes his turn at a transition relevance place (i.e. associated with an attributable silence). It will be useful to see how the conversational partners handle such silences, if they do occur. The balance of major and minimal turns between the conversationalists will also indicate who is bearing the main load of the conversation.

Analysis: Topic management.

Justification for selection: As AC is reporting difficulty following conversation, topic change may be particularly difficult for him. Examination of whether he experiences any difficulty orienting to new topics will be informative.

Results of the conversation analyses

> Now read through the findings of the analyses undertaken.

Conversational data collected: A recording was made between AC and his daughter in AC's home. The audio taperecorder was set up and left for the conversational partners to turn on at the start of one of the daughter's frequent visits.

Analysis of repair patterns: As predicted from his phonological impairment, AC made a large number of self-repairs in the conversation, the majority involving phonemic paraphasias, for example:

(Target: 'topiary')
AC [kɔpəri] that's [kɔpəri] that's a good word for it [kə kɔpjəri]

(Target: 'tapering'? 'shaping'?)
AC I'll get that as I'm going [ʃɛɪp ʃɛip ʃɛipərɪŋ] in to it yes

Although AC did not always manage to achieve the correct phonological target, his self-repair attempts usually gave enough information for his daughter to understand what the target was and, after a brief demonstration of the understanding that she had reached, the conversation moved on without requiring extensive collaborative work. The following example shows how AC supplements phonological attempts with semantic information to assist his conversational partner:

AC in the [ɒld] the er (0:7) [ɒl ɒli obɪtɛnli] the hhh (0.5) not like university like we used <to have>
CP <a poly>technic?
AC mm yes

On some occasions, when his daughter repeated a word that he was having difficulty with, AC attempted to repeat it but made further phonological errors. This had the effect of extending the collaborative repair as his daughter provided further models for him to attempt the target.

AC used editing terms extensively in his conversational turns, the majority of which occurred by themselves. Repetition of whole phrases and multiple repetitions of words occurred. Although pauses within his turns did occur, these were either filled or were predominantly less than 1 second. Despite some word-finding difficulties, therefore, AC was effective in holding on to his conversational turn and gaining more time to deal with processing difficulties. For example:

AC but I also did it at Newcastle hhh and er and and and erm in Middlesborough

In the 10 minutes of conversation that were transcribed, 16 collaborative repair sequences initiated on AC's turns were identified. These predominantly involved clarification of either a phonological error or a lexical selection error, an example of which is provided below:

AC so you had a good meeting [gə] you had a good afternoon then?
CP weekend?
AC weekend yeah
CP yes mhm yesterday we spent pulling the lounge to bits

As seen in this example, all the collaborative repair sequences were resolved quickly with AC's daughter checking her understanding of the problematic item. In all cases she was correct, and so the conversation could continue without further repair work.

AC was observed to request clarification of his daughter's turns on 12 occasions. These could reflect the comprehension deficit that he reports. All except two were quickly resolved, with his daughter providing clarification and the conversation continuing. There were two sequences, however, where it was clear that AC had not reached the correct understanding but his daughter let it go, an example of which is given below. AC does not reach the understanding that the journey took two and a half hours, and after three clarifications of this, his daughter lets his understanding that it took two hours go.

AC and how long did it take you to get today (.) the time?
CP to get down there?
AC mm

CP   two and a half hours
AC   half an hour
CP   two and a half
AC   two two
CP   two hours and a \<half\>
AC   \<two\> two hours
CP   aha

Analysis of turn-taking: AC was able to handle turn-taking well. As discussed above, in relation to self-repair, he showed the ability to hold the conversational floor through his strategies of repetitions and filled pauses. As a result, the proportion of major turns was evenly distributed between AC and his daughter (53: 47).

Analysis of topic management: There was no evidence in the conversation of difficulties in topic management. AC was able to orient to changes of topic when they were introduced by his daughter.

Planning initial intervention

From the findings of these assessment results it is proposed that AC's predominant impairment lies at the level of the phonological assembly buffer, with other possible lexical retrieval and auditory comprehension problems. Conversation analysis indicates that AC nevertheless participates effectively in communication in a one-to-one domestic situation, and takes a full share of the conversational load. A number of repair strategies have been noted. What therapy would you derive from the findings of the psycholinguistic assessments and the conversation analysis?

Our suggestions for initial intervention

> Now that you have thought about some possible interventions, compare them with our suggestions. Remember that these are only tentative ideas and may differ from yours. Both your and our ideas may be appropriate. The important issue is that intervention should be motivated by theoretical principles.

An initial decision to be made is whether any intervention is required, and whether any such intervention should take the form of direct therapy aimed at remediating what seems to be AC's major difficulty in assembling words, or should be focused on facilitating communication through reducing the conversational impact of this difficulty. AC's involvement in this decision will be essential.

Although AC's difficulties now make his conversational exchanges different from what could be presumed to be his pre-morbid patterns, interaction between him and his daughter was not significantly impeded, and he carried a full share of the conversational load. There were examples, however, of the flow of conversation being interrupted by AC's continuing attempts to seek a correct phonological realisation even when the meaning of the target word had been conveyed. AC's attention is clearly focused on self-repair, and the value of this could perhaps be discussed with him and his conversational partners, in order to consider whether unnecessary extensions of repair sequences should be reduced. Further conversational samples may help to clarify the wisdom of taking this approach. AC also makes relatively little use of circumlocutions, and this might be encouraged as a strategy which would enable his familiar conversational partners to effect other-repairs and/or continue the flow without interruption. Use of advice booklets, such as those described in Lesser and Algar (1995) and Booth et al. (1999) could be considered, in order to foster the insights of AC and his family into both his psycholinguistic difficulties and the effective use of conversational strategies.

Assistance through direct therapy for his phonological problems may also help to reduce AC's need to engage in self-repairs. Such direct therapy could capitalise on AC's superior performance when he reads words rather than having to find them in his lexicon or concentrate on their phonological form through repetition. AC also clearly finds monosyllabic productions relatively easy. Using both these assets, AC could be encouraged to segment written poly-syllabic words and build their pronunciation up part by part. The effects of frequency noted in the assessments suggest that repeated practice could improve performance through increasing the level of activity of these items in the lexicon. As a preliminary to such direct therapy, however, it would be desirable to undertake a more detailed analysis of AC's phonemic paraphasias. For instance, the extent to which the putative form of the word is accessed could be investigated through analysis of the number of syllables, the frequency with which the initial phoneme or initial syllable is correctly accessed, the pattern of lexical stress and the effect of cueing with word fragments. Therapy aimed at remediation of phonological assembly is little described in the literature, although De Partz (1995) has described a segmentation strategy aimed at a deficit of the graphemic assembly buffer. One example of a (pre-psycholinguistic) personal approach to a phonological assembly disorder identified as 'conduction aphasia' is in Simmons (1983). She describes the therapy task continuum she used with a specific patient, utilising a Base-10 format for monitoring progression. This consisted of asking him to repeat and read monosyllabic nouns and then verbs. Two-second delays were introduced, and then sentences of the format 'You verb a noun'. No evaluation, however, of the success of this programme is reported.

There are also other questions to be asked about the level of AC's auditory comprehension, especially given the evidence of impairment of this from the conversation analysis (see next page).

Developing the hypotheses

> Remember that the results of assessment (and of intervention) feed back into developing the hypotheses you initially made. There may also be gaps in your interpretation, which the results have revealed. Write down what further investigations you might wish to consider to develop your hypotheses, some of which may depend on AC's response to therapy.

Our suggestions for developing the hypotheses

> Now read through the suggestions that we have made and compare them with your own.

As outlined in our suggestions for intervention, a number of further investigations of AC's phonemic paraphasias could help to clarify the nature of his assembly disorder, and the extent to which the phonological output lexicon is also involved. A modality comparison of form retrieval in speech and in writing (or oral spelling) could also help to provide more evidence as to the involvement of more central aspects of lexical processing. To clarify this, further information is also needed about AC's abilities to retrieve words for insertion into sentence frames in comparison with the naming of isolated items. An analysis of elicited connected speech could be used for this, where the target lexical items could be identified by using picture description or narratives of well-known stories.

The psycholinguistic assessments reported here have provided little information on AC's reported problems with auditory comprehension. A hypothesised impairment of access from an intact phonological input lexicon to an intact semantic system was proposed from the results of the synonym judgement test, which could underlie some problems of comprehension. It is feasible, however, that AC might have difficulties which implicate syntactic abilities and/or the mapping of thematic roles, and assessments which examine these would be helpful. Possible assessments that include pragmatically reversible sentences could be used, such as PALPA 55 *Auditory sentence comprehension* or the Test for the Reception of Grammar (TROG).

It was also proposed that AC's poorer performance on the auditory synonym judgement assessment could be explained by a reduced span in auditory short-term memory. This could be examined through PALPA 60 *Noun verb pointing span*. A further explanation for the discrepancy between AC's good auditory comprehension on formal tests and impaired immediate comprehension in conversation could be in his ability to focus his attention on constrained activities, with greater difficulty in coping with the many variables of an open-ended conversation. Assessment with the Test of Everyday Attention (Robertson et al., 1994) would allow us to explore this.

Conclusions

Through the six example cases you have just worked with, we have tried to illustrate the principles of applying cognitive neuropsychology (CN) and conversation analysis (CA) to the understanding of how aphasia presents in individuals. As the cases are real ones, and the data are the ones that were actually collected, we hope that aphasia therapists will find this of practical use in clinical work. As you will have noted, we have been eclectic in our choice of tests. To some extent this reflects the resources available in our clinics, though it also acknowledges the present deficiencies in cognitive neuropsychological assessments, despite the advances over the last decade. For example, in Case 1 (Mr AR) we have used subtests from the Aphasia Screening Test (Whurr, 1981) to examine the patient's ability to do simple matching, and in Case 3 (Mrs JA), we have used subtests from the BDAE (Goodglass and Kaplan, 1983) to examine the ability to imitate melody and rhythm.

In working through the cases you may well have found yourselves choosing different tests from those we have presented. Looking back on the cases ourselves we have noted where, with hindsight (and more time for thought under the pressures of clinical work), we also would have chosen different tests. We can but hope that you will have learned not only from your own practice with the workbook but from our faults. The cases in this workbook therefore have a different flavour from the finely honed ones which appear in the journal literature. Not all aphasic patients have the resilience to endure the prolonged testing which can be a feature of these published research cases.

Need for converging evidence

Although we are aware of the need for economy in testing, we must nevertheless emphasise the need to use assessments to provide converging evidence. One assessment is not sufficient to reveal the level of breakdown, although it may show that preceding levels must be at least partly functional when the patient succeeds in a task which draws on them as well as the targeted level. For example, AR's success (Case 1) in auditory lexical decision implied that phonological analysis and hearing were intact and did not need to be scrutinised. In contrast, in Case 6 (Mr AC), a number of tests were necessary to establish that his major difficulty was in phonological assembly. Complementing cognitive neuropsychological assessment with CA provides another source of evidence to check on the validity of interpretation of a disorder.

A major deficiency in our psycholinguistic presentation of the cases is the lack of information about sentence processing. The same principles of assessment that we have illustrated, however, apply to this as to the processing of single words, and the practice of assessing the processing of sentences is well illustrated, with materials and examples, in a recently published handbook (Marshall et al., 1999). As Whitworth (1995) has demonstrated, studying a patient's use of words in sentences can be illuminating as to the nature of anomia, usually considered as a disorder in retrieving single words. Whitworth showed that it is possible to distinguish between people whose word-retrieval difficulties in sentences are due to sentence level processes (management of thematic roles) and ones which are due to lexical difficulties as such.

Although we have used tests of reading in most of our cases (Cases 1, 2, 4 and 6) and of writing in three (Cases 3, 4 and 5), we have used these different modalities as tests of the centrality of the putative disorder, rather than as examinations of reading and writing in their own right. This has been deliberate on our part, since the analysis of the dyslexias and dysgraphias, both as 'pure' disorders and as part of aphasia, is a major study on its own. PALPA provides a number of materials which are helpful in assessing dyslexia, and distinguishing at which processing levels the reading disorder can be detected. Amongst the many texts on dyslexia and dysgraphia, a readable one is Ellis (1984).

In the final three cases of the workbook, converging evidence from both CN and CA is provided, allowing an exploration of the impact of the individual's cognitive neuropsychological assets and deficits on conversational interaction. Knowledge of the loci of deficits informs an understanding of what is happening in the conversation, for example, in Case 5 (Mrs JN), the presence of a central semantic impairment informed the understanding of her production of conversational turns with non-specific referring expressions. The CA also informs the CN investigations. For example, for Case 4 (Mrs EM), the severity of word-finding difficulties that she experienced in conversation led us to suggest that assessment of thematic role processing (which plays an important role in word finding at a sentence level) should be undertaken. Perhaps most importantly, the strength of converging evidence from CN and CA emerges in the use of the assessment results to inform therapy.

Moving from assessment to therapy: an integrated approach

From the results that we have presented and your interpretation of the cases' loci of disorder (and its impact on conversation for the final three cases), we hope that you will have found a logical link to how therapy might be developed. The cognitive neuropsychological approach has traditionally been associated with impairment-focused therapy in which remediation of, or compensation for, the underlying language processing deficit is addressed. This link can certainly be seen in the cases we have presented. For example, 'reactivation' of lost ability was suggested for Cases 1 and 5 through re-establishing semantic knowledge, while, for Case 4, use of retained orthographic information to compensate for impaired access to the phonological output lexicon was proposed. We also hope to have illustrated, however, that CN assessment findings also inform communication-focused therapy. CN assessment identifies what abilities may be drawn upon in developing communication strategies. For example, in Case 1, AR's better access to semantics through the written modality led to the suggestion that development of a communication book could assist in compensating for impaired comprehension.

The final three cases of the book included converging evidence from CA as well as from CN. These findings were also found to have implications for both impairment-focused and communication-focused therapy. CA allowed an examination of whether the deficits identified from CN assessments compromised interactional ability, thus assisting in the identification of the most valid targets for impairment-focused therapy. For example for Case 6, whereas manifestation of a deficit compromising the phonological output buffer was seen in conversation, interaction was not significantly impeded, thus bringing into question the need for impairment-focused therapy. This contrasts to the situation for Case 4, for whom an impairment involving the phonological output lexicon severely compromised her participation in interaction, suggesting the need for impairment-focused therapy.

CA assessment findings also have implications for planning compensation-focused therapy. While, as outlined above, CN assessment findings can inform this approach to therapy, CA provides the extra dimension of focusing on the role of both conversational partners in the collaborative construction of conversation. As exemplified in Case 4, the comparison that was made between a conversation with her relative and with her therapist introduced a further dimension. Specifically, while predictions can be made from cognitive neuropsychological assessments with respect to the impact that deficits will have on interaction (and these were made in the first three cases of the book for which CA assessment findings were not provided), the precise impact will also be influenced by the conversational partner's interactional strategies. Identification from CA assessment of precisely the strategies that the person with aphasia and his or her conversational partner are using and their outcome provides a rational motivation for therapy focused on the development and modification of strategies.

In conclusion, we hope that in working through the cases in this book that you have gained an insight into the complementary strengths that CN and CA offer and the potential that an integration of the two approaches has for the provision of rationally motivated aphasia therapy.

References

Ahlsen A (1985) Discourse patterns in aphasia. Gothenburg Monographs in Linguistics, 5. Department of Linguistics, University of Gothenburg.

Atkinson JM, Drew P (1979) Order in Court: the Organisation of Verbal Interaction in Judicial Settings. London: Macmillan.

Barry C (1996) Testing cognitive neuropsychology. Cognitive Neuropsychology 13: 1201–6.

Behrmann M, Lieberthal T (1989) Category-specific treatment of a lexical-semantic deficit: a single case study of global aphasia. British Journal of Disorders of Communication 24: 281–99.

Behrmann M, McLeod J (1995) Rehabilitation for pure alexia: efficacy of therapy and implications for models of normal word recognition. Neuropsychological Rehabilitation 5: 149–80.

Berndt RS, Mitchum CC (1994) Approaches to the rehabilitation of 'phonological assembly': elaborating the model of nonlexical reading. In Riddoch MJ, Humphreys GW (eds) Cognitive Neuropsychology and Cognitive Rehabilitation. Hove: Lawrence Erlbaum Associates.

Best W, Howard D, Bruce C, Gatehouse C (1997) Cueing the words: a single case study of treatments for anomia. Neuropsychological Rehabilitation 7: 105–41.

Bishop DVM (1983) Test for the Reception of Grammar. Oxford: MRC and Thomas Leach.

Booth S, Perkins L (1999) The use of conversation analysis to guide individualised advice to carers and to evaluate change in aphasia: a case study. Aphasiology 13 (4&5): 289–81.

Booth S, Paterson W, Wilson G (1999) Personalised Advice Booklets for Aphasia. Glasgow: Glasgow Royal Infirmary.

Bryan K (1989) Right Hemisphere Battery. Leicester: Far Communications.

Buerk F, Franklin S, Howard D. (1997) Self-monitoring therapy for a client with conduction aphasia. British Aphasiology Society Biennial International Conference, Manchester.

Butterworth B (1979) Hesitation and the production of verbal paraphasias and neologisms in jargonaphasia. Brain and Language 8: 133–61.

Button G, Casey N (1984) Generating topic: the use of topic initial elicitors. In Atkinson JM, Heritage J (eds) Structures of Social Action: Studies in Social Action. Cambridge: Cambridge University Press.

Byng S (1995) What is aphasia therapy? In Code C, Muller D (eds) Treatment of Aphasia: From Theory to Practice. London: Whurr.

Byng S, Nickels L, Black M (1994) Replicating therapy for mapping deficits in agrammatism: remapping the deficit? Aphasiology 8: 315–41.

Caramazza A. (1989) Cognitive neuropsychology and rehabilitation: an unfulfilled promise? In Seron X, Deloche G (eds) Cognitive Approaches in Neuropsychological Rehabilitation. Hillsdale, NJ: Lawrence Erlbaum.

Caramazza A. (1998) The interpretation of semantic category-specific deficits: what do they reveal about the organization of conceptual knowledge in the brain? Neurocase 4: 265–272.

Carlomagno S, Van Eeckhout P, Blasi V, Belin P, Samson Y, Deloche G (1997) The impact of functional neuroimaging methods on the development of a theory for cognitive remediation. Neuropsychological Rehabilitation 7: 295–326.

Christensen AL (1974) Luria's Neuropsychological Investigation. Copenhagen: Munksgaard.

Clark HH, Schaefer EF (1987) Collaborating on contributions to conversations. Language and Cognitive Processes 2: 19–41.

Clark HH, Schaefer EF (1989) Contributing to discourse. Cognitive Science 13: 259–94.

Code C (1987) Language, Aphasia and the Right Hemisphere. Chichester: Wiley.

Coltheart M (1989) Aphasia therapy research: a single-case study approach. In Code C, Muller D (eds) Aphasia Therapy, 2nd edn. London: Cole and Whurr.

Conway N (1990) Repair in the conversations of two dysphasics with members of their families. Unpublished BSc dissertation, University of Newcastle upon Tyne.

Couper-Kuhlen E (1992) Contextualizing discourse: the prosody of interactive repair. In Auer P, Di Luzio A (eds) The Contextualization of Language. Amsterdam: Benjamins.

Crockford C, Lesser R (1994) Assessing functional communication in aphasia: clinical utility and the time demands of three methods. European Journal of Disorders of Communication 29: 55–72.

Dabul BL (1986) Apraxia Battery for Adults. Oregon: C.C. Publications.

Davidoff J, De Bleser R (1993) Optic aphasia: a review of past studies and reappraisal. Aphasiology 7: 135–54.

Davis GA, Wilcox MJ (1985) Adult Aphasia Rehabilitation. San Diego, CA: College Hill Press.

De Bleser R, Cholewa J, Stadie N, Tabatabaie S (1997) LeMo, an expert system for single case assessment of word processing impairments in aphasic patients. Neuropsychological Rehabilitation 7: 339–65.

De Partz MP (1995) Deficit of the graphemic buffer: effects of a written lexical segmentation strategy. Neuropsychological Rehabilitation 5: 129–47

DeRenzi E, Pieczuro A, Vignolo LA (1966) Oral apraxia and aphasia. Cortex 2: 50–73.

Duffy RJ, Duffy JR (1984) New England Pantomime Tests. Tigard, OR: C.C. Publications.

Edwards S, Garman M (1989) Case study of a fluent aphasic: the relation between linguistic assessment and therapeutic intervention. In Grunwell P, James A (eds) The Functional Evaluation of Language Disorders. London: Croom Helm.

Ellis AW (1984) Reading, Writing and Dyslexia: A Cognitive Analysis. London: Lawrence Erlbaum.

Ellis AW, Franklin S, Crerar A (1994) Cognitive neuropsychology and the remediation of disorders of spoken language. In Riddoch MJ, Humphreys GW (eds) Cognitive Neuropsychology and Cognitive Rehabilitation. Hove: Lawrence Erlbaum Associates.

Fasold R (1990) The Sociolinguistics of Language. Oxford: Blackwell.

Fleming C (1989) An analysis of the communication strategies employed by aphasics when conversing with other aphasics. Unpublished BSc dissertation, University of Newcastle upon Tyne.

Francis WN, Kučera H (1982) Frequency Analysis of English Usage: Lexicon and Grammar. Boston, MA: Houghton Mifflin.

Franklin S (1989) Dissociations in auditory word comprehension: evidence from nine fluent aphasic patients. Aphasiology 3: 189–207.

Franklin S (1997) Designing single case treatment studies for aphasic patients. Neuropsychological Rehabilitation 7: 401–18.

Franklin S, Howard D, Patterson K (1995) Abstract word anomia. Cognitive Neuropsychology 12: 549–66

Franklin S, Turner J, Ellis AW (1992) The ADA Comprehension Battery. London: Action for Dysphasic Adults.

Franklin S, Turner J, Lambon Ralph MA, Morris J, Bailey PJ (1996) A distinctive case of word meaning deafness? Cognitive Neuropsychology 13: 1139–62.

Garfinkel H (1972) Remarks on ethnomethodology. In Gumperz JJ, Hymes DH (eds) Directions in Sociolinguistics. New York: Holt, Rinehart and Winston.

Garrett KL, Beukelman DR, Low-Morrow D (1989) A comprehensive augmentative communication system for an adult with Broca's aphasia. Augmentative and Alternative Communication 5: 55–64.

Gilchrist ID, Humphreys GW, Riddoch MJ (1996) Grouping and extinction: evidence for low-level modulation of visual selection. Cognitive Neuropsychology 13: 1223–49.

Goffman E (1955) On face work. Psychiatry 18: 213–31.

Goodglass H, Kaplan E (1983) The Assessment of Aphasia and Related Disorders (Boston Diagnostic Aphasia Examination, BDAE). Philadelphia: Lea and Febiger.

Goodman R, Caramazza A (1985) The Johns Hopkins University Dysgraphia Battery. The Johns Hopkins University, Baltimore, MD.

Grayson E, Franklin S, Hilton R (1997) Early intervention in a case of jargon aphasia: efficacy of language comprehension therapy. European Journal of Disorders of Communication 32: 257–76.

Green G (1982) Assessment and treatment of the adult with severe aphasia: aiming for functional generalisation. Australian Journal of Human Communication Disorders 10: 11–23.

Greenwald ML, Raymer AM, Richardson ME, Rothi LJG (1995) Contrasting treatments for severe impairments of picture naming. Neuropsychological Rehabilitation 5: 17–49.

Helm-Estabrooks N, Fitzpatrick PM, Barresi B (1982) Visual action therapy for global aphasia. Journal of Speech and Hearing Disorders 47: 385–9.

Heritage J, Atkinson JM (1984) Introduction. In Atkinson JM, Heritage J (eds) Structures of Social Action: Studies in Social Action. Cambridge: Cambridge University Press.

Hillis AE (1992) The role of models of language processing in rehabilitation of language impairments. Aphasiology 7: 5–26.

Hillis AE, Caramazza A (1994) Theories of lexical processing and rehabilitation of lexical deficits. In Riddoch MJ, Humphreys GW (eds) Cognitive Neuropsychology and Cognitive Rehabilitation. Hove: Lawrence Erlbaum Associates.

Howard D, Hatfield FM (1987) Aphasia Therapy: Historical and Contemporary Issues. Hove: Lawrence Erlbaum Associates.

Howard D, Patterson K (1992) Pyramids and Palm Trees. Bury St Edmunds: Thames Valley Test Co.

Howard D, Patterson K, Franklin S, Orchard-Lisle V, Morton J (1985) The treatment of word retrieval deficits in aphasia: a comparison of two therapy methods. Brain 108, 817–29.

Howard D, Patterson K, Wise R, Brown WD, Friston K, Weiller C, Frakowiak R (1992) The cortical localization of the lexicons: positron emission tomography evidence. Brain 115: 1769–92.

Humphreys GW, Riddoch MJ (1987) To See But Not to See: A Case Study of Visual Agnosia. Hove: Lawrence Erlbaum Associates.

Huskins S (1989) Treatment of articulatory apraxia in aphasic patients. In Code C, Muller D (eds) Aphasia Therapy, 2nd edn. London: Whurr.

Jefferson G (1984) On the organization of laughter in the talk about troubles. In Atkinson JM, Heritage J (eds) Structures of Social Action: Studies in Social Action. Cambridge: Cambridge University Press.

Jefferson G (1987) On exposed and embedded correction in conversation. In Button G, Lee JRE (eds) Talk and Social Organisation. Clevedon: Multilingual Matters.

Jones EV (1984) Word order processing in aphasia: effect of verb semantics. In Rose FC (ed.) Advances in Neurology 42: Progress in Aphasiology. New York: Raven.

Kagan A (1995) Revealing the competence of aphasic adults through conversation: a challenge to health professionals. Topics in Stroke Rehabilitation 2: 15–28.

Kagan A, Gailey GF (1993) Functional is not enough: training conversational partners for aphasic adults. In Holland AL, Forbes MM (eds) Aphasia Treatment: World Perspectives. London: Chapman Hall.

Kaplan E, Goodglass H, Weintraub S (1983) Boston Naming Test. Philadelphia, PA: Lea and Febiger.

Kay J, Lesser R, Coltheart M (1992) Psycholinguistic Assessments of Language Processing in Aphasia (PALPA). Hove: Lawrence Erlbaum.

Kay J, Lesser R, Coltheart M (1996) Psycholinguistic assessments of language processing in aphasia (PALPA): an introduction. Aphasiology 10: 159–215.

Kent RD (1998) Neuroimaging studies of brain activation for language, with an emphasis on functional Magnetic Resonance Imaging: a review. Folia Phoniatrica et Logopaedica 50: 291–304.

Kopelman M, Wilson B, Baddeley A (1990) Autobiographical Memory Interview. Bury St Edmunds: Thames Valley Test Co.

Lambon Ralph MA, Sage K, Ellis AW (1996) Word meaning blindness: a new form of acquired dyslexia. Cognitive Neuropsychology 13: 617–39.

LaPointe LL (1984) Sequential treatment of split lists. In Rosenbek JC, McNeil MR, Aronson AE (eds) Apraxia of Speech. San Diego, CA: College Hill Press.

Le Dorze G (1990) Protocole d'evaluation des troubles lexico-semantiques. Version experimentale. Quebec: University of Montreal.

Le Dorze G, Boulay N, Gaudreau J, Brassard C (1994) The contrasting effects of a semantic versus a formal-semantic technique for the facilitation of naming in a case of anomia. Aphasiology 8: 127–41.

Lesser R (1990) Superior oral to written spelling: evidence for separate buffers. Cognitive Neuropsychology 7: 347–66.

Lesser R (1993) Aphasia therapy. In Blanken G, Dittman J, Grimm H, Marshall JC, Wallesch CW (eds) Linguistic Disorders and Pathologies: An International Handbook. Berlin: Walter de Gruyter.

Lesser R (1995) Making psycholinguistic assessments accessible. In Code C, Muller D (eds) Treatment of Aphasia: From Theory to Practice. London: Whurr.

Lesser R, Algar L (1995) Towards combining the cognitive neuropsychological and the pragmatic in aphasia therapy. Neuropsychological Rehabilitation 5: 67–92.

Lesser R, Milroy L (1993) Linguistics and Aphasia: Psycholinguistic and Pragmatic Aspects of Intervention. London: Longman.

Linebaugh CW (1983) Treatment of anomic aphasia. In Perkins WH (ed.) Language Handicaps in Adults. New York: Thieme-Stratton.

Lowell S, Beeson P, Holland AL (1995) The efficacy of semantic cueing procedures on naming performance of adults with aphasia. American Journal of Speech-Language Pathology 4: 383–94.

Lyon J, Helm-Estabrooks N (1987) Drawing: its communicative significance for expressively restricted adults. Topics in Language Disorders 8: 61–7.

Lyon J, Sims E (1989) Drawing: its use as a communicative aid with aphasic and normal adults. In Prescott T (ed.) Clinical Aphasiology, vol.18. Boston, MA: College Hill Press.

Lyon JG (1989) Communicative partners: their value in re-establishing communication with aphasic adults. In Prescott T (ed.) Clinical Aphasiology Conference Proceedings. San Diego, CA: College Hill Press.

Manochiopinig S, Sheard C, Reed VA (1992) Pragmatic assessment in adult aphasia: a clinical review. Aphasiology 6: 519–33.

Marshall J, Pound C, White-Thomson M, Pring T (1990) The use of picture/word matching tasks to assist word retrieval in aphasic patients. Aphasiology 4: 167–84.

Marshall J, Black M, Byng S (1999) Working with Sentences: A Handbook for Aphasia Therapists (in The Sentence Processing Resource Pack). Bicester: Winslow.

Miceli G, Capasso R, Caramazza A (1994) The interaction of lexical and sub-lexical processes in reading, writing and repetition. Report 94-6 of the Cognitive Neuropsychology Laboratory, Dartmouth College, Hanover, NH.

Miceli G, Laudanna A, Caramazza A (1991) Batteria per l'analisi dei deficit afasici. Volume 1. Milano: Berdata.

Miller N (1989) Strategies of language use in assessment and therapy for acquired dysphasia. In Grunwell P, James A (eds) The Functional Evaluation of Language Disorders. London: Croom Helm.

Milroy L, Perkins L (1992) Repair strategies in aphasic discourse: towards a collaborative model. Clinical Linguistics and Phonetics 6: 27–40.

Mitchum CC, Berndt RS (1995) The cognitive neuropsychological approach to treatment of language disorders. Neuropsychological Rehabilitation 5: 1–16.

Morris J, Franklin S (1995) Assessment and remediation of a speech discrimination deficit in a dysphasic patient. In Perkins M, and Howard S (eds) Case Studies in Clinical Linguistics. London: Whurr.

Morris J, Franklin S, Ellis AW, Turner JE, Bailey PJ (1996) Remediating a speech perception deficit in an aphasic patient. Aphasiology 10: 137–58.

Nettleton J, Lesser R (1991) Therapy for naming difficulties in aphasia: application of a cognitive neuropsychological model. Journal of Neurolinguistics 6: 139–57.

Newhoff M, Bugbee J, Ferreira A (1981) A change of PACE: spouses as treatment targets. In Brookshire R (ed.) Clinical Aphasiology Conference Proceedings. Minneapolis: BRK.

Nicholas M, Helm-Estabrooks N (1990) Aphasia. Seminars in Speech and Language 11: 135–44.

Patterson K, Purell C, Morton J (1989) Facilitation of word retrieval in aphasia. In Code C, Muller D (eds) Aphasia Therapy, 2nd edn. London: Whurr.

Perkins L (1995a) Applying conversation analysis to aphasia: clinical implications and analytic issues. European Journal of Disorders of Communication 30: 372–83.

Perkins L (1995b) An exploration of the impact of psycholinguistic impairments on conversational ability in aphasia. International Journal of Psycholinguistics 11: 167-88.

Perkins L (in press) Negotiating repair in aphasic conversation: interactional issues. In Goodwin C (ed.) The Pragmatic Life of Bain-Damaged Patients. Cambridge: Cambridge University Press.

Perkins L, Crisp J (1997) Exploring CA as an assessment tool for aphasia. Paper presented at International Conference on Disorder and Order in Talk: Conversation Analysis and Communication Disorders, London.

Perkins L, Lesser R, Milroy L (1998) Conversation Analysis and Aphasia: Theoretical and Clinical Applications. End of Award Report on ESRC Project R000236456. Swindon: ESRC.

Perkins L, Crisp J, Walshaw D (1999) Exploring Conversation Analysis as an assessment tool for aphasia: the issue of reliability. Aphasiology 13 (4&5): 283–303.

Reisberg D, McLean J, Goldfield A (1987) Easy to hear but hard to understand: a lip-reading advantage with intact auditory stimuli. In Dodd B, Campbell R (eds) Hearing by Eye: The Psychology of Lip-reading. Hove: Lawrence Erlbaum Associates.

Robertson IH, Ward T, Ridgeway V, Nimmo-Smith I (1994) Test of Everyday Attention. Bury St Edmunds: Thames Valley Test Co.

Sacks H (1984) On doing 'being ordinary'. In Atkinson JM, Heritage J (eds) Structures of Social Action: Studies in Social Action. Cambridge: Cambridge University Press.

Sacks H (1992) Lectures on Conversation. Oxford: Blackwell.

Sacks H, Schegloff E, Jefferson G (1974) Simplest systematics for the organisation of turntaking in conversation. Language 50: 696–735.

Schegloff EA (1979) The relevance of repair to syntax-for-conversation. In Talmy Givon (ed.) Syntax and Semantics 12: Discourse and Syntax. New York: Academic Press.

Schegloff EA (1982) Discourse as an interactional achievement: some uses of 'uh huh' and other things that come between sentences. In Tannen D (ed.) Georgetown Roundtable on Language and Linguistics 93. Georgetown: University Press.

Schegloff EA (1987) Some sources of misunderstanding in talk-in-interaction. Linguistics 25: 201–18.

Schegloff EA (1988) Discourse as an interactional achievement II: An exercise in Conversation Analysis. In Tannen D (ed.) Linguistics in Context: Connecting Observation and Understanding. Norwood: Ablex.

Schegloff EA (1992) Repair after next turn: the last structurally provided defense of intersubjectivity in conversation. American Journal of Sociology 97: 1295–345.

Schegloff EA (1993) Reflections on quantification in the study of conversation. Research on Language and Social Interaction 26: 99–128.

Schegloff E, Jefferson G, Sacks H (1977) The preference for self-correction in the organisation of repair in conversation. Language 53: 361–82.

Schiffrin D (1988) Conversation analysis. In Frederick J (ed.) Linguistics: The Cambridge Survey. Cambridge: Cambridge University Press.

Seidenberg M (1988) Cognitive neuropsychology and language: the state of the art. Cognitive Neuropsychology 5: 403–26.

Seron X, Deloche G, Bastard,V, Chassin G, Hermand N (1979) Word finding difficulties and learning transfer in aphasic patients. Cortex 15: 149–55.

Shallice T, Glasspool DW, Houghton G (1995) Can neuropsychological evidence inform connectionist modelling? Analysis of spelling. Language and Cognitive Processes 10: 195–225.

Siegel S (1956) Non-parametric Statistics for the Behavioral Sciences. Tokyo: McGraw-Hill, pp 63–7.

Simmons NN (1983) Treatment of conduction aphasia. In Perkins WH (ed.) Language Handicaps in Adults. New York: Thieme-Stratton.

Snodgrass JG, Vanderwort M (1980) A standardized set of 260 pictures: norms for naming agreement, familiarity and visual complexity. Journal of Experimental Psychology: Human Learning and Memory 6: 174–215.

Sparks RW, Deck JW (1986) Melodic intonation therapy. In Chapey R (ed.) Language Intervention Strategies in Adult Aphasia, 2nd edn. Baltimore, MD: Williams and Wilkins.

Square-Storer P (1989) Traditional therapies for apraxia of speech - reviewed and rationalised. In Square-Storer P (ed.) Acquired Apraxia of Speech in Aphasic Adults: Theoretical and Clinical Issues. London: Taylor and Francis.

Square-Storer P, Hayden D (1989) PROMPT treatment. In Square-Storer P (ed.) Acquired Apraxia of Speech in Aphasic Adults: Theoretical and Clinical Issues. London: Taylor and Francis.

Taskmaster Resources (1997) Category Cards, Sets 1 and 2. Morris Road, Leicester LE2 6BR: Taskmaster Ltd.

Thompson J, Enderby P (1979) Is all your Schuell really necessary? British Journal of Disorders of Communication 14: 195–201.

Warrington EK, James M (1991) Visual Object and Space Perception Battery. Bury St Edmunds: Thames Valley Test Co.

Wertz RT (1984) Response to treatment in patients with apraxia of speech. In Rosenbek JC, McNeil MR, Aronson AE (eds) Apraxia of Speech. San Diego, CA: College Hill Press.

Wertz RT, LaPointe LL, Rosenbek JC (1984) Apraxia of Speech in Adults: The Disorder and its Management. Orlando, FL: Grune and Stratton.

Whiting S, Lincoln N, Bhavani G, Cockburn J (1985) Rivermead Perceptual Assessment Battery. Windsor: NFER-Nelson.

Whitworth A (1994) Thematic role assignment in word-retrieval deficits in aphasia. Unpublished PhD thesis, University of Newcastle upon Tyne.

Whitworth A (1995) Characterising thematic role assignment in aphasic sentence production: procedures for elicited and spontaneous output. European Journal of Disorders of Communication 30: 384–99.

Whitworth A (1996) Thematic Roles in Production (TRIP): an assessment of word retrieval at the sentence level. London: Whurr.

Whitworth A, Perkins L, Lesser R (1997) Conversation Analysis Profile for People with Aphasia (CAPPA). London: Whurr.

Whurr R (1981) Aphasia Screening Test. London: Whurr.

Wilkinson R (1995) Doing 'being ordinary': aphasia as a problem of interaction. In Kersner M, Pepe S (eds) Work in Progress, vol. 5. Department of Human Communication Science: University College London.

Willmes K (1995) Aphasia therapy research; some psychometric considerations and statistical methods for the single-case study approach. In Code C, Muller D (eds) Treatment of Aphasia: From Theory to Practice. London: Whurr.

Wilson B, Cockburn J, Baddeley A (1985) Rivermead Behavioural Memory Test. Bury St Edmunds: Thames Valley Test Co.

York Cognitive Neuropsychology Research Group (1996) How to Help with Specific Language Problems: a Set of Eight Booklets. 1 Royal Street, London SE1 7LL: Action for Dysphasic Adults.

Appendix A

Guidelines on evaluation of direct intervention for aphasia in a clinical setting

This is not presented as an ideal model, but as a practical way of attempting a rough-and-ready evaluation of direct therapy within a relatively short span (e.g. a student's clinical placement). It does not include psychosocial facilitation, functional communication and other important aspects of intervention.

1. Decide from your initial assessments whether it is appropriate to use direct therapy for any aspect of the patient's language processing and, if so, what aspect to target and what materials to use. Look in the therapy literature for examples of papers describing such therapy (such as are mentioned in the case studies in this workbook), and replicate this therapy if appropriate, with or without modifications.

2. See if there is another aspect of the patient's language disabilities that you do not intend to work on immediately, and which would not be predicted to be affected by the therapy you are planning. This will act as a control measure (Control Task C) for pre-therapy and post-therapy tests, to see whether the patient is recovering generally regardless of therapy.

3. Randomly divide the therapy materials you are going to use into two comparable sets, i.e. one for use in therapy (Set T, the Treatment Set) and one not to be used and therefore to act as an untreated set to test for generalisation of the therapy (Set U, the Untreated Set). (You might predict generalisation for some therapies, such as semantic therapy for naming, and not for others, such as learning some spelling lists.) Make sure the two sets, T and U, are of equivalent difficulty, i.e. that the patient has had the same degree of success with each.

4. Get baseline scores for the patient on all the treatment and control materials. To make the baselines more reliable, repeat the baseline assessments at least once (you might be able to do this at the beginning and end of one session or over two sessions).

5. Give the therapy over as many sessions as you can or as many sessions as are appropriate.

6. Retest the patient on all the three tasks (Set T, Set U and Set C).

7. For each set, test whether the 'after' scores are now significantly different from the baseline 'before' scores, using the McNemar Test for the Significance of Changes (Siegel, 1956). An easy way to do this with minimal calculations is to use Table A1, for which we are indebted to David Howard. For each 'before' and 'after' pair of scores (i.e. on Set T, Set U and Set C), tot up how many items were better on the second occasion and how many were worse. Look at the table and find the place where these two figures meet. If the number there is in bold print you can say that the probability of getting that result by chance is less than 5 in a 100.

These are only the bare bones of evaluation, but they should give you a start with putting this into practice. You could incorporate into this scheme, for suitable cases, a possible measure of some generalisation to functional communication by conversation analyses before and after treatment. You could incorporate 'before' and 'after' ratings by a carer. You could (if time permitted) use a 'multiple baseline paradigm', by switching half-way through to therapy for what had been the control set of language materials in your first therapy. This would give you comparisons of treatment and no treatment periods for both aspects, and you could test whether any changes in scores coincided with the different episodes of treatment and non-treatment.

Worked example

DW has difficulty in pronouncing polysyllabic words and produces prolonged phonemic paraphasias. A preliminary assessment, using a psycholinguistic model, suggests that his main difficulty lies at the level of the phonological assembly buffer. It is decided to treat this by a programme of reading aloud of polysyllabic words, in which he is taught the strategy of breaking them up into individual syllables and then recombining them.

Before therapy he is assessed on the reading aloud of a list of 50 polysyllabic words. These are then randomly divided into two sets of 25, with the constraint that each set includes an equal number of items on which he has made errors. These will be used as Set T (to be worked on in therapy) and Set U (to be left untreated). It is predicted that, if he learns the strategy, he will be able to apply it generally, and that there will therefore be improvement on the untreated set as well as on the treated set. His 'before' score on each set is 4 out of 25.

The control task C needs to be one which, according to the model, does not involve the phonological assembly buffer, and which will not be expected to improve through the planned treatment. It is decided to use as the control task another process with which he has some difficulty, i.e. writing words to dictation, and to use only words which have exceptional spellings, so that a lexical route must be used in writing them rather than a phoneme-to-grapheme route through the phonological assembly buffer to the graphemic assembly buffer. His 'before' score on this control list is 8 out of 25.

After the treatment, his scores are: Set T 14 out of 25; Set U 10 out of 25, Set C 12 out of 25. These are made up as follows:

Set T items 'after' scores

worse 2	correct again 2
wrong again 9	better 12

Set U items 'after' scores

worse 1	correct again 3
wrong again 14	better 7

Set C items 'after' scores

worse 5	correct again 3
wrong again 8	better 9

For the McNemar Test for the Significance of Changes, all we need note are the scores which show changes, i.e. are 'worse' or 'better'. Using Table A1 we see that for Set T, with two items worse (see left hand column) and 12 items better (see numbers across the top), the probability is 0.006. There are therefore only six chances in 1000 of getting this result by chance, i.e. this makes it highly probable that a real change has taken place.

For Set U, with one item worse and seven items better, the probability is 0.035. This is also significant, but with 35 chances in 1000 of getting this result by chance. It supports the prediction that there would be some generalisation of the work done on the treated set to the untreated set.

For Set C, the control set, with five items worse and nine items better, the probability is 0.212. This is not significant. This result could support the claim that the improvement in Sets T and U is not due just to spontaneous recovery or the fact that someone has been showing an interest, though we cannot be sure that it is not due to the difference between the nature of the two tasks employed. We could follow this up by now giving therapy for the Set C task, and then reassessing on Sets T, U and C. This would tell us whether the writing task also showed improvement in association with therapy, and also whether the improvement on Sets T and U has been maintained.

We would also want to test whether the therapy has led to another kind of generalisation, generalisation to different contexts. We therefore need to test whether DW now makes fewer phonemic paraphasias in word-finding for naming and in conversation. To do this we would also need to have obtained scores on DW's naming and samples of conversation before starting the therapy.

Table A1: One-tailed probabilities when the number of items given across the top are better on the second occasion, and the number of items in the left-hand column are worse

Number of items better on second test

	1	2	3	4	5	6	7	8	9	10	11	12	13	14	15	16	17	18	19	20	21	22	23	24	25
0	.500	.250	.125	.062	**0.31**	**.016**	**.008**	**.004**	**.002**	**.001**	**.000**	**.000**	**.000**	**.000**	**.000**	**.000**	**.000**	**.000**	**.000**	**.000**	**.000**	**.000**	**.000**	**.000**	**.000**
1		.500	.312	.187	.109	0.62	**.035**	**.020**	**0.11**	**.006**	**.003**	**.002**	**.001**	**.000**	**.000**	**.000**	**.000**	**.000**	**.000**	**.000**	**.000**	**.000**	**.000**	**.000**	**.000**
2			.500	.344	.227	.145	.090	.055	**.033**	**.019**	**.011**	**.006**	**.004**	**.002**	**.001**	**.001**	**.000**	**.000**	**.000**	**.000**	**.000**	**.000**	**.000**	**.000**	**.000**
3				.500	.363	.254	.172	.113	.073	**.046**	**.029**	**.018**	**.011**	**.006**	**.004**	**.002**	**.001**	**.001**	**.000**	**.000**	**.000**	**.000**	**.000**	**.000**	**.000**
4					.500	.377	.274	.194	.133	.090	.059	**.038**	**.025**	**.015**	**.010**	**.006**	**.004**	**.002**	**.001**	**.001**	**.000**	**.000**	**.000**	**.000**	**.000**
5						.500	.387	.291	.212	.151	.105	.072	**.048**	**.032**	**.021**	**.013**	**.008**	**.005**	**.003**	**.002**	**.001**	**.001**	**.000**	**.000**	**.000**
6							.500	.395	.304	.227	.166	.119	.084	.058	**.039**	**.026**	**.017**	**.011**	**.007**	**.005**	**.003**	**.002**	**.001**	**.001**	**.000**
7								.500	.402	.315	.240	.180	.132	.095	.067	**.047**	**.032**	**.022**	**.014**	**.010**	**.006**	**.004**	**.003**	**.002**	**.001**
8									.500	.407	.324	.252	.192	.143	.105	.076	.054	**.038**	**.026**	**.018**	**.012**	**.008**	**.005**	**.003**	**.002**
9										.500	.412	.332	.262	.202	.154	.115	.084	.061	**.044**	**.031**	**.021**	**.015**	**.010**	**.007**	**.005**
10											.500	.416	.339	.271	.212	.163	.124	.092	.068	**.049**	**.035**	**.025**	**.018**	**.012**	**.008**
11												.500	.419	.345	.279	.221	.172	.132	.100	.075	.055	**.040**	**.029**	**.020**	**.014**
12													.500	.423	.351	.286	.229	.181	.141	.108	.081	.061	**.045**	**.033**	**.024**
13														.500	.425	.356	.292	.237	.189	.148	.115	.088	.066	**.049**	**.036**
14															.500	.428	.360	.298	.243	.196	.155	.121	.094	.072	.054
15																.500	.430	.364	.304	.250	.203	.162	.128	.100	.077
16																	.500	.432	.368	.309	.256	.209	.168	.134	.106
17]																		.500	.434	.371	.314	.261	.215	.174	.140
18																			.500	.436	.375	.318	.266	.220	.180
19																				.500	.437	.378	.322	.271	.226
20																					.500	.439	.380	.326	.276
21																						.500	.440	.383	.329
22																							.500	.441	.358
23																								.500	.443
24																									.500

Probability values significant at P<0.05 are in bold.

Appendix B

Aphasia tests referred to in the case studies

ADA (Action for Dysphasic Adults) Comprehension Battery (ADACB) (Franklin, Turner and Ellis, 1992)

- P1 and P2 *Non-word minimal pairs*. The person with aphasia is asked to listen to 40 recorded pairs of consonant-vowel-consonant (CVC) syllables, and decide whether these represent the same items or not. The initial or final phonemes differ by one or two features. In P1 the items are spoken by the same person, and may therefore only require acoustic discrimination. In P2 one item in each pair is spoken by a man and one by a woman, so that the match must be made at a phonological level.

- P3 *Real word minimal pairs*. This 40-item test uses the same procedure as P1, but with real words. It can help to establish whether people with impaired phonemic perception are aided by the use of lexical information.

- L1 *Lexical decision test*. This 160-item test (given over two sessions) consists of recorded words and non-words varied by length (<4, >4 phonemes), imageability (high, low) and frequency (high, low). The task is to judge whether each item is a real word in English.

- S1 *Synonym judgements*. This uses 160 recorded word pairs, half of which have the same or similar meanings. The items are controlled for imageability and frequency. The task is to judge whether the two words mean (almost) the same thing.

- S2 and S2Wr *Spoken word–picture matching* and *Written word–picture matching*. Both these tests consist of 66 words, recorded in the case of S2 and presented in printed form in the case of S2Wr. They are accompanied by sets of four shaded drawings of objects; each set comprises a representation of the target word, two unrelated distractors and a distractor, which is phonologically or semantically or both phonologically and semantically related to the target word.

Aphasia Screening Test (Whurr, 1981)

- Matching subtests A1–8. In these five-item subtests the person with aphasia is asked to match visual materials (subtests A1–4) or written materials (subtests A5–8). The visual materials comprise line drawings of objects, colours, shapes and actual objects. The written materials comprise numbers, letters, words and sentences.
- Reading subtests A9–11. These assess reading comprehension by asking the person to match five words and five sentences to pictures and to follow five simple written commands.
- Auditory Comprehension subtests A13–17. In these five-item subtests the individual is asked to match spoken words to pictures, spoken colour names to coloured patches and spoken words to numbers, letters and printed words.

Apraxia Battery for Adults (Dabul, 1979)

There are six subtests in this battery:

- Diadochokinetic rate, in which the individual attempts to repeat syllables rapidly over 3 seconds.
- Repetition of words, with their length increased by the addition of one then two morphemes.
- Ten items testing limb apraxia (e.g. make a fist) and 10 testing oral apraxia (e.g. stick out your tongue).
- Timed naming of pictures, where the target word is polysyllabic.
- Repeating three times the words used in subtest 4.
- Based on spontaneous speech or reading aloud, an inventory of the features of 'articulatory apraxia' shown by the person.

Boston Diagnostic Aphasia Examination (BDAE) (Goodglass and Kaplan, 1983)

- The *auditory comprehension* section consists of four subtests, concerned respectively with matching words with pictures or symbols (line drawings of objects or actions, letters, colours, shapes and numbers), body-part identification, executing commands and giving yes/no answers to sentences and questions about paragraphs.

- The *oral agility* section consists of six items where the person with aphasia is asked to make repeated mouth movements and six similar items using word repetitions.
- In the *recitation, singing and rhythm* section the person is asked to recite automatised matter such as nursery rhymes, sing a familiar song and imitate tapped rhythms.
- There are two *repetition tests*, one using only words, the other using phrases distinguished as of high or low probability.
- *Naming* is tested in part through confrontation naming of line drawings of objects and actions, colours, letters, shapes and body parts, and through responsive naming to questions.
- *Reading comprehension* is tested in part through selection of one printed word from four to match a spoken word, and selection of a line drawing of an object, action, shape, number or colour for a printed word.

Boston Naming Test (Kaplan, Goodglass and Weintraub, 1983)

Sixty line drawings represent words of roughly decreasing frequency, from 'bed' to 'abacus'. If the person with aphasia gives a response that indicates misperception of the drawing, a set cue as to meaning is supplied. If the individual fails to name within 20 seconds, or says he or she does not know the word, a set phonemic cue is given.

Conversation Analysis Profile for People with Aphasia (CAPPA) (Whitworth, Perkins and Lesser, 1997)

This profile consists of a structured interview to be conducted with the person with aphasia and/or his or her key conversational partner, a method of analysis of a 10-minute sample of unscripted conversation recorded between them, and a summary profile that combines the interview and the conversational sample. Section A of the interview asks questions about a range of conversational management features, as well as seeking a description of what strategies are used to cope with them. Section B of the interview elicits a comparison of pre-morbid and current interactional styles and opportunities. The method for analysis of conversation looks for evidence of the same conversational management features explored in the interview, and examines the strategies being employed to deal with any difficulties that emerge. The summary profile provides an opportunity to compare information from the two sources.

Kay Naming Test (revised, unpublished)

This 75-item test is a precursor of PALPA 54. It uses line drawings representing words controlled for three levels of frequency (high, medium, low). It can be used for oral and written naming to provide a comparison of modalities.

Mono-poly Picture Naming Test (Lesser, unpublished)

Twenty line drawings representing monosyllabic words are matched for word frequency and manmade/living nature with 20 representing three- or four-syllable words. All words are of low frequency, but within this low band three levels are distinguished, i.e. 'high' occurring more than three times in Francis and Kuçera (1982), 'medium' occurring once or twice and 'low' not occurring in this database. There is a greater number of clusters in the monosyllabic words than in the polysyllabic; this bias reduces the likelihood that more errors in naming polysyllabic items are due to articulatory difficulties as such.

New England Pantomime Tests (Duffy and Duffy, 1984)

The three tests are: Pantomime Recognition (Forms A and B), Pantomime Expression and Pantomime Referential Abilities. In the first, the tester mimes 46 or 40 items and the individual is asked to select from four line drawings, one of which is a semantic distractor and two of which are unrelated distractors. In the second, the person with aphasia demonstrates the functions of 23 pictured items. In the third, the person is asked to mime a message so that a receiver can make a correct choice from four pictures which include a visual distractor, a distractor associated with the same location in space or body and an unrelated distractor.

Psycholinguistic Assessments of Language Processing in Aphasia (PALPA) (Kay, Lesser and Coltheart (1992)

1. *Same-different discrimination using non-word minimal pairs.* The 72 CVC non-words in this test are contrasted by initial, final or reversed initial-final (metathetic) places in the syllable. They are also balanced for different types of articulatory contrast: voice, place, manner.
2. *Same-different discrimination using word minimal pairs.* This 72-item test using CVC words is controlled for the same factors as test 1. In addition, word frequency is controlled, with half of the 'same' pairs being of high frequency and half low.

3. *Minimal pair discrimination requiring written word selection.* This uses the same words as in test 2, but the response is to tick the spoken word from printed pairs.

4. *Minimal pair discrimination requiring picture selection.* Forty spoken CVC words are used, each with three line drawings shown. The names of the drawings for two of the distractors differ from the target's name by either one or two+ distinctive features. Initial, final and metathetic contrasts are used, controlled for voice, place and manner of articulation. For half the sets the minimal pair distractor is of lower frequency than the target, while for the other half it is of similar or higher frequency.

5. *Imageability and frequency auditory lexical decision.* Eighty words of one, two or three syllables are spoken, mixed with 80 non-words of similar lengths. The words are controlled for imageability (high/low) and frequency (high/low). The task is to indicate whether they are real words or not.

7. *Syllable length repetition.* Twenty-four words (eight each of one, two and three syllables) are spoken for the individual to repeat. The sets of words are matched for frequency, imageability and morphemic complexity.

8. *Non-word repetition.* Thirty non-words (10 each of one, two and three syllables) are spoken for the individual to repeat. Phoneme length is constant across the sets.

9. *Imageability and frequency repetition.* A list of 80 words and 80 non-words is used for repetition, either as separate lists or one mixed list. The words are an expanded set of those used in tests 5, 25 and 31 for lexical decision and oral reading. The words are controlled for frequency and imageability.

25. *Imageability and frequency visual lexical decision.* Sixty printed words are mixed with 60 non-words, for the person to tick the real words recognised. The words are controlled for imageability and frequency and, within sub-groups, for number of letters, syllables, morphemes and grammatical class. Non-words are derived from the words by changing one or two letters.

27. *Visual lexical decision and spelling-sound regularity.* In a mixed list 15 regular words, 15 exceptionally spelled words, 15 pseudohomophones (e.g. gote) and 15 non-words which are not homophonous with real words are presented in printed form for the person to tick the words which he or she recognises.

30. *Oral reading: syllable length.* Eighteen five-letter printed words of from one, two or three syllables are presented for reading aloud.

31. *Oral reading: imageability and frequency*. The task is to read aloud 80 words. The words are the same as those in test 5.

35. *Spelling-sound regularity and reading*. Thirty regularly spelled and 30 exception words are mixed and presented in printed form for reading aloud.

36. *Non-word reading*. Twenty-four monosyllabic non-words are presented in printed form for reading aloud. The non-words are in four sets increasing in length from three to six letters.

39. *Spelling to dictation: letter length*. Six monosyllabic words each of three, four, five and six letters are dictated.

40. *Imageability × frequency spelling*. A 40-item list of words for dictation, a subset of those used to test oral reading in PALPA 31.

47. *Spoken word–picture matching*. A 40-item test, in which the individual has to select one from five line drawings to match a heard word. The distractors are either closely or distantly semantically related, or visually related or unrelated. Half of the close semantic distractors also are visually similar (e.g. 'cat' for 'dog').

48. *Written word–picture matching*. The reading version of PALPA 47, with the target word printed in the centre of the five drawings.

49. *Auditory synonym judgements*. A 60-item test, controlled for imageability of the items (high/low). The person is asked to indicate whether pairs of heard words mean 'nearly the same thing'.

50. *Written synonym judgements*. The reading version of PALPA 49, the response being to tick pairs of words which mean nearly the same thing.

51. *Word semantic association*. This 30-item written test is in two parts, using words of high and low imageability respectively. The person is shown an underlined word and asked to tick which of four words is closest in meaning to it.

53. *Picture naming × oral reading, repetition and written spelling*. Forty line drawings are provided for naming. The written forms of the names are controlled for regular/exceptional spelling. This version is therefore also informative for reading aloud (a printed list for reading is provided), naming through writing and written spelling. To complete the modality comparisons, it can also be used for spoken repetition.

54. *Picture naming × frequency*. Sixty words are provided for picture naming, controlled for frequency (high, medium, low). Pictures are not provided, but should be selected from Snodgrass and Vanderwart (1980).

55. *Auditory sentence comprehension.* Sixty spoken sentences are presented with sets of three line drawings representing the target and two distractors, one of which is a grammatical contrast such as reversal of subject and object, the other using a lexical distractor. Twenty of the sentences are reversible, 16 are non-reversible, 16 use gapped sentences such as 'The girl's suggesting/asking what to eat', and eight use converse relations such as 'The man's taking/giving the prize.

56. *Written sentence comprehension.* This uses the same materials as PALPA 55 in a different order, and with the sentence printed at the bottom of each page of three drawings.

60. *Pointing span for noun–verb sequences.* This test of short-term auditory verbal memory uses a picture pointing response to sets of spoken words which imitate SV, SVO, SV+SV structures etc. The items increase in number from two to six. Four of the eight pictures represent nouns and four verbs.

Pyramids and Palm Trees Test (three-picture version) (Howard and Patterson, 1992)

In this 52-item test, a picture is presented with a choice of two pictures from which to select the associate. Different types of conceptual/semantic information are used, e.g. perceptual as in associating a curtain with a window rather than a door, and knowledge of the world as in associating a pyramid with a palm tree rather than a pine tree. The test can also be presented in five other versions, i.e. with three written words, and in various combinations of pictures and written and spoken words.

Shortened (British) form of the Minnesota Test for the Differential Diagnosis of Aphasia (Thompson and Enderby, 1979)

Section A of this test, 'Auditory Disturbances', comprises nine subtests with five items each. They are:

1. matching words to pictures
2. discriminating between paired monosyllabic words differing in one distinctive feature
3. recognizing the names of letters

4. pointing to items named serially in a composite picture
5. understanding sentences (yes/no answers)
6. following commands
7. understanding a paragraph (yes/no answers)
8. repeating digits
9. repeating sentences.

The naming and repetition subtests are part of Section C, 'Speech and Language Disturbances'. They comprise repetition of five monosyllabic words and five phrases, and naming five days of the week and five line drawings.

Test for the Reception of Grammar (TROG) (Bishop, 1983)

This test is unique among the ones listed here in that it was originally designed for children and uses sets of four coloured pictures. It is now commonly used for screening sentence comprehension in aphasic adults. Its 80 items increase in difficulty from single words (three blocks of four items) to sentences (17 blocks of four items), with discriminations involving negatives, locative prepositions, plurals, comparative adjectives, passives and embeddings. There is an optional vocabulary check which uses cards with eight drawings from which to select an object name, shape name, verb or adjective.

Thematic Roles in Production (TRIP) (Whitworth, 1996)

This test compares the ability to produce isolated nouns as the names of pictures with the ability to produce the same nouns in sentences as descriptions of pictures. The sentences involve one-argument ('The baby's waving'), then two-argument ('The woman's lifting the baby'), then three-argument structures ('The woman's giving the shell to the baby'). The nouns occur as agents, or as patients in two-argument structures or as patients in the second argument of three-argument structures. All the items are first described by the tester so that a model answer is heard before the test begins. The test is divided into two similar parts, comprising 39 items and 41 items respectively.

Appendix C

Transcription conventions for conversational data

(0.0)	Pauses or gaps in tenths of seconds.
(x syll.)	Number of inaudible syllables.
( )	Uncertain passages of transcript.
[ ]	Broad phonetic transcription.
hhh	Audible out-breath.
'hhh	Audible in-breath.
= =	Latched utterances with no gap.
{ }	Non-verbal activity denoted between brackets, including laughter.
< >	Parts of utterances which are produced in overlap.
T1, T2, ...	Numbered turns.

Worksheets for photocopying

Your initial hypotheses

> Using the information given in the case description, consider the possible loci of the impairments. Given the limited information that you have, you may have several tentative hypotheses. What is the justification for each of the hypotheses? What further information would you require to confirm or reject each of these?

The difficulties compromise the _____

_____

Justification for this is that _____

_____

_____

_____

_____

_____

_____

The difficulties compromise the _____

_____

Justification for this is that _____

_____

_____

_____

_____

_____

The difficulties compromise the _____

_____

_____

Justification for this is that

The difficulties compromise the

Justification for this is that

The difficulties compromise the

Justification for this is that

What other factors need to be taken into consideration in planning assessments?

Your selection of assessments

> Now that you have some initial hypotheses about the loci of impairments, plan the types of assessment tasks that you would employ to test out your hypotheses. We have provided spaces for several assessments, but this does not mean that we expect you to use the exact number. You will find that selection of one assessment will be influenced by the potential findings of previous ones carried out.

Assessment

_____

Justification for selection

_____
_____
_____
_____
_____
_____

Assessment

_____

Justification for selection

_____
_____
_____
_____
_____
_____

Assessment

_____
_____

Justification for selection

Assessment

Justification for selection

Assessment

Justification for selection

Your interpretation of the results of the assessments

What do the assessment results mean? Map out your hypotheses of the locus or loci of the deficits based on these findings, using the diagram of the model. Indicate also what processes seem to be preserved and which levels you are uncertain about from the assessment results so far. Note down the justification in support of your hypotheses.

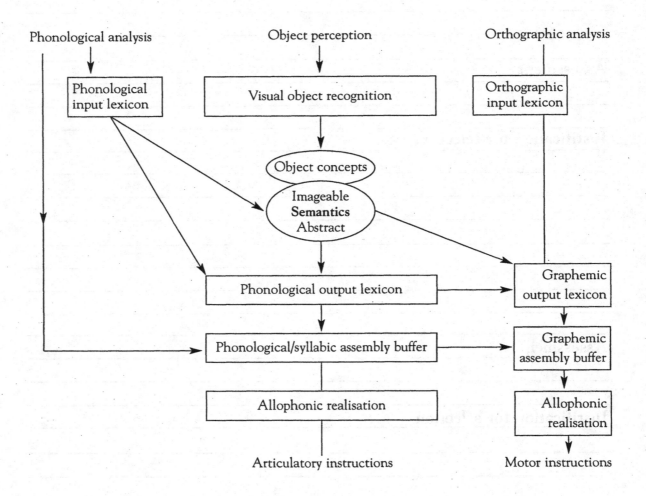

Justification for hypotheses

_____

_____

_____

_____

Conversation analysis: selecting parameters for assessment

We will ask you shortly what inferences for therapy you might draw from the psycholinguistic findings. Meanwhile from the results of the cognitive neuropsychological assessment and the information given in the case description, consider what analyses of conversation you would like to undertake to gain information to guide therapy.

Conversational data to be collected

Analysis

Justification for selection

Analysis

Justification for selection

Planning intervention

What initial approach to therapy would you derive from the assessment results?

Developing the hypotheses

Remember that the results of assessment (and of intervention) feed back into developing the hypotheses you initially made. There may also be gaps in your interpretation, which the results have revealed. Use this page to write down what further investigations you might wish to consider to develop your hypotheses, some of which may depend on response to therapy.

Index